MEDITERRANEAN DIET
THE AUSTRALIAN WAY

taste.com.au

MEDITERRANEAN DIET
THE AUSTRALIAN WAY

HarperCollins*Publishers*

harpercollins.com.au

CONTENTS

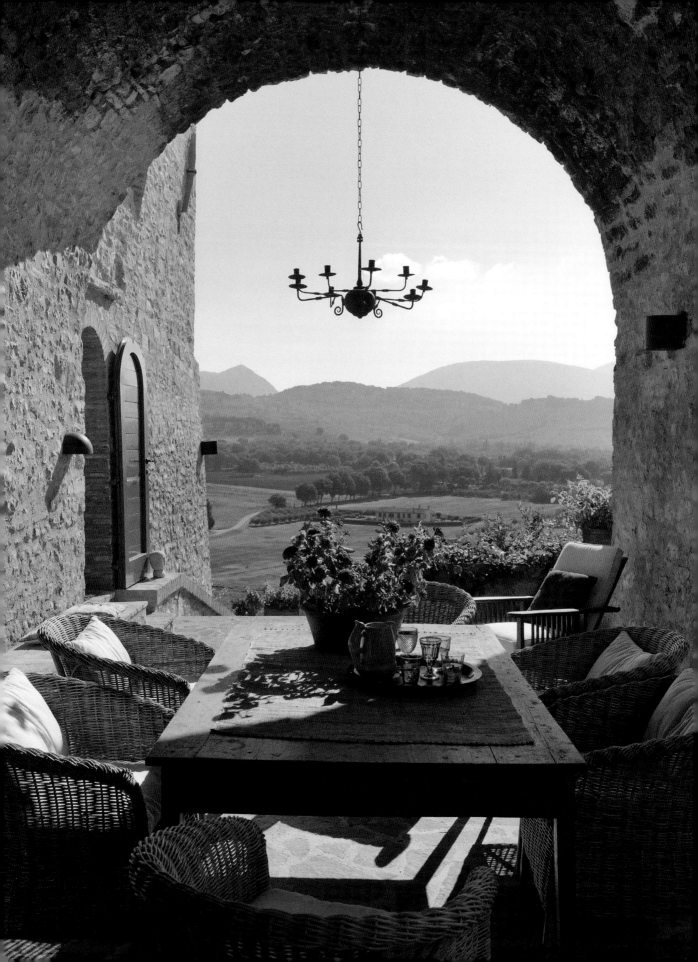

HELLO!

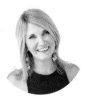

How much do we love the Med diet? Let us count the ways. It's delicious and nutritious. It's easy, affordable and good for the planet, with roots interwoven, over thousands of years, with the life of peasants. And did we mention it's roundly considered by experts as the world's #1 healthiest diet?

Yet, there's another reason to love the Mediterranean diet that we don't talk about enough. And that's how well it translates into the Australian context. Certainly we have everything at our fingertips that the diet calls for in fresh, plentiful abundance, from vegetables and fruits, to wholegrains and legumes, and fresh omega-rich fish. And it doesn't stop there. This diet is as much a way of living as it is a way of eating. Social connection and getting together around the table is 'baked' in as part of it.

Mediterranean Diet: The Australian Way, finally, for the first time, brings together our ultimate collection of taste.com.au recipes that fit the Mediterranean diet criteria. But it's more than just a cookbook, it's a complete guide to use every day for every meal and snack, to unleash the full power of this diet and transform your health. There's enough here for a lifetime – and according to the science, you'll have a lot more of that if you follow this diet.

Best of all, this is a diet for food lovers who also want to eat well without deprivation (that's me!). Nothing's off the menu – it's always about balance. You've got to hand it to the Mediterranean peoples of old. This really is a diet for life.

Enjoy!

Brodee

BRODEE MYERS,
EDITOR-IN-CHIEF

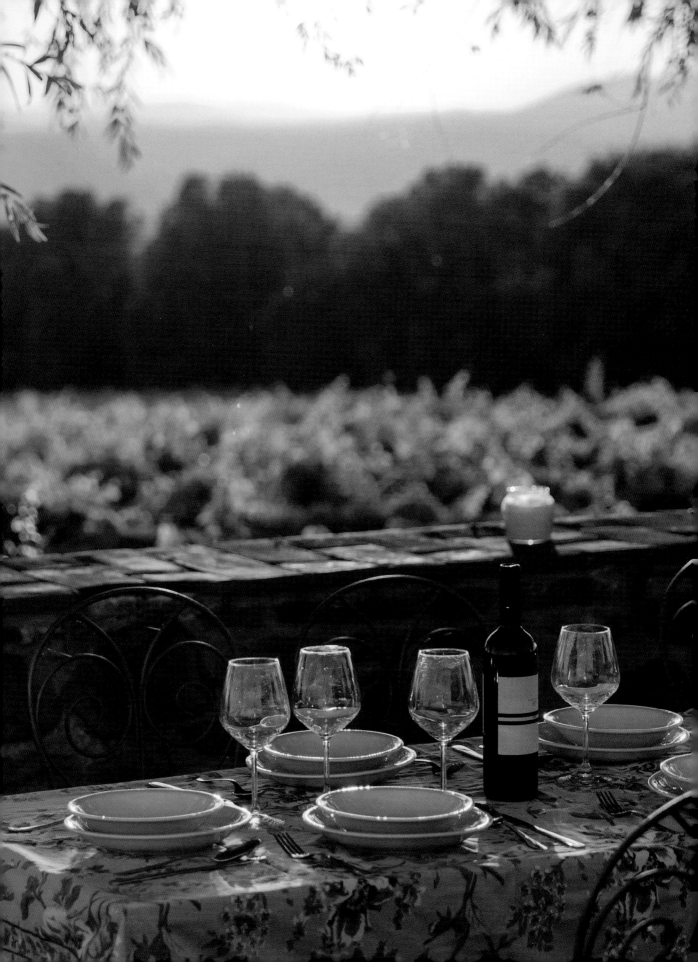

MED ON THE MENU

Considered the best in the world, the Mediterranean diet offers mighty health benefits. Nutritionist Chrissy Freer explains why Australia is a great place to eat and live this way.

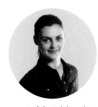

When it comes to diets, the traditional Mediterranean diet stands head and shoulders above the rest. Nutritionists and scientists the world over agree. What other diet can you think of that's recognised on the UNESCO Intangible Cultural Heritage List for its significance and value to humanity?

When we say 'traditional' Mediterranean diet, we're referring to a diet with origins that go back thousands of years to the dietary habits of regional communities around the wide geographical region known as the Mediterranean Basin. Countries such as Greece, Italy, Portugal, Spain, Croatia, Cyprus and Morocco, that surround the Mediterranean Sea. Each has its own ingredients and flavour profiles. But what they share are common dietary principles and characteristics.

What has evolved from these traditional dietary habits is now defined as the Mediterranean dietary pattern, with a strong focus on natural whole foods. It's described as 'predominately plant based' on account of the high prevalence of fresh fruit and vegetables, wholegrains, legumes, and nuts and seeds. Other key features include extra virgin olive oil and moderate-to-high intakes of fish and seafood captured fresh from the sea.

Consumed in lesser amounts are foods such as eggs, poultry and dairy (typically Greek yoghurt and feta), while red meat, meat products and processed foods are limited. The focus is on seasonal and local produce.

However, the Mediterranean diet is not just a way of eating, it's a way of life. It is the literal meaning of the Greek word *diaita*. In fact, it encompasses a whole lifestyle. Adequate rest and physical activity, eating meals as a family and living as part of an active, engaged community are also important parts of living this way.

The Mediterranean diet is in stark contrast to the modern Western dietary ▶

Australia is fortunate to have an abundant and diverse range of fresh produce, and seafood is plentiful. It's an ideal place to embrace the Mediterranean way of eating.

patterns and lifestyle, which is typified by high intakes of processed foods, low intakes of fruit and vegetables, low physical activity levels and often a disconnect with community. We know that these modern traits are also risk factors for poor health, with rates of chronic diseases – such as obesity, type 2 diabetes, cardiovascular disease and fatty liver – rapidly escalating in Western countries.

THE DIET WITHIN AUSTRALIA

What makes this diet so valuable? It's based on food and lifestyle habits that are flexible enough to translate into our real world and everyday living.

While it is not possible to replicate the millennia of history, culture or seasonal produce grown in the Mediterranean, there is much we can learn from this traditional dietary pattern. In a modern Australia, the underlying core principles can be adopted to promote overall health and wellbeing.

Australia, being an island with a unique geographical location, is fortunate to have an abundant and diverse range of fresh produce, and seafood is plentiful.

We can enjoy a Mediterranean diet with an Aussie twist. Diversity and variety of plant-based foods is recognised as being pivotal to good health and nutrition, making Australia an ideal place to embrace the Mediterranean way of eating.

WHY IT'S GREAT

This is one of the most scientifically researched diets globally. Experts have found several health benefits associated with adhering to this dietary pattern.

Based mainly on plant foods, it has an impressive nutrient profile: rich in dietary fibre and other beneficial plant compounds, such as polyphenols and antioxidants, as well as good fats (monounsaturated and omega 3 fatty acids), while low in processed sugars and saturated fat.

The overall cardiometabolic benefits are notable: associated with a reduced risk of cardiovascular disease, type 2 diabetes, high blood pressure and cholesterol.

It can play a protective role against certain cancers, including breast, prostate, liver and stomach, and is known to assist weight management. ▶

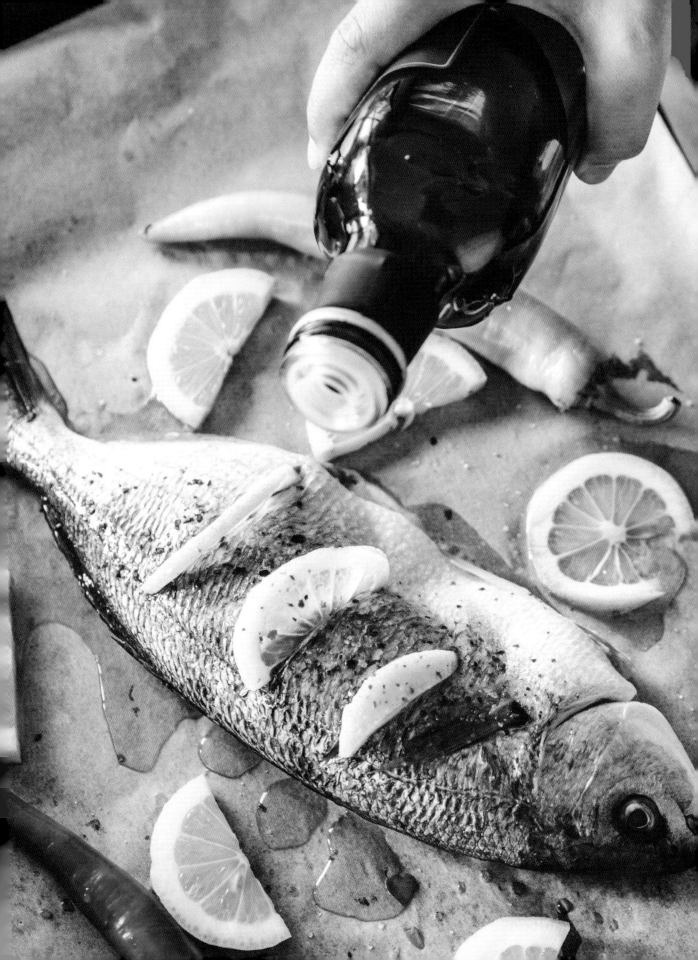

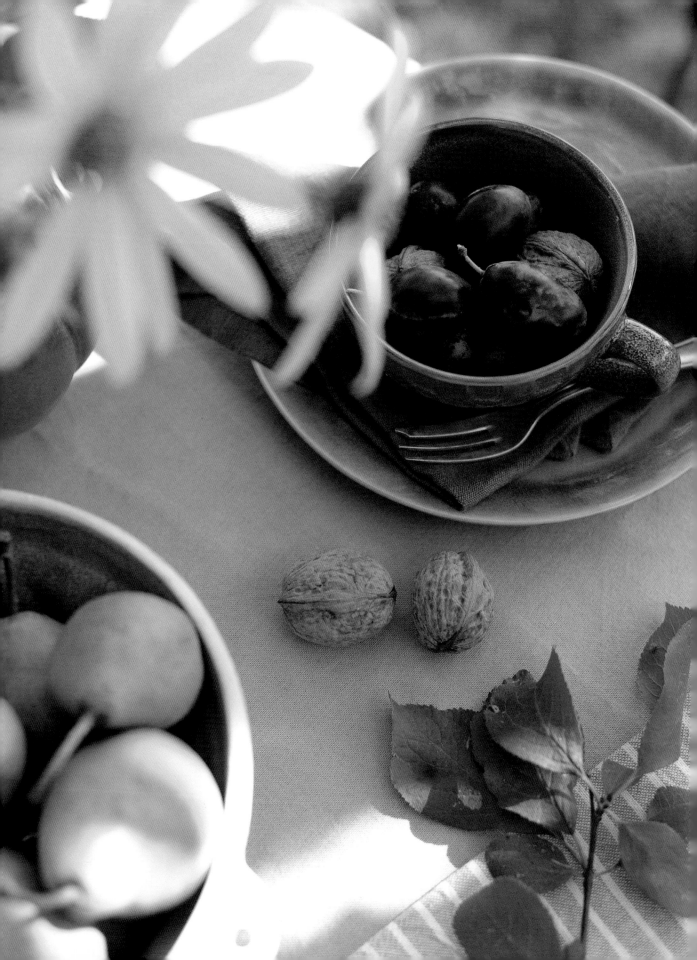

Its high content of monounsaturated and omega 3 fatty acids and other anti-inflammatory plant compounds can help lower chronic inflammation and may assist inflammatory conditions, such as arthritis.

Also on the list is improved mental health, with recent research demonstrating the diet may reduce the risk of depression and dementia, and even improve cognition.

HOW TO GET STARTED

No food or food group is excluded. It's more about how often and how much of different foods should be consumed.

Food to eat more

Being predominantly plant based, fresh fruit and vegetables should form the foundation of all meals, while grains and cereals (mainly in their wholegrain form) are also important. For example, wholemeal couscous, wholegrain sourdough bread, wholemeal pasta, barley, burghul and quinoa.

Aim for diversity in your fruit and veg intake with different types and colours. This assures a wide range of beneficial plant compounds, such as polyphenols and antioxidants. Use extra virgin olive oil for cooking, salad dressings and drizzling over vegetables. This provides healthy monounsaturated fats. Use onion, garlic, fresh herbs and spices in abundance to add flavour.

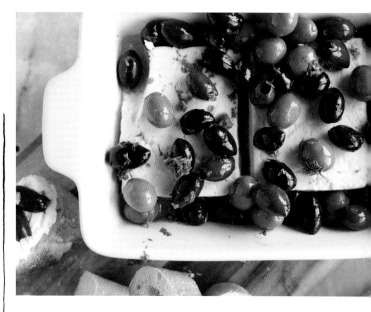

Food to eat regularly

Eat a variety of protein sources, including plant-based proteins, such as legumes – think lentils, chickpeas and black beans. Add to salads, braises, casseroles and grain-based dishes, such as pilaf. Snack on nuts and seeds or sprinkle over salads or yoghurt and fruit.

When choosing animal proteins, go for more seafood at least twice a week. Eggs, white meats and dairy (Greek yoghurt, feta and low-fat milk are good choices) can still be enjoyed in moderation.

Food to eat less often

Eat red meat and processed meats, such as salami and bacon, less often and in smaller portions. Reduce processed grains, sweets and ultra-processed foods. Opt for fruit, yoghurt and occasionally enjoy homemade desserts that are fruit- and wholegrain-based.

THE
Mediterranean diet
PYRAMID

Use this as your handy, at-a-glance guide to the
Mediterranean diet's optimal plan for eating and living.

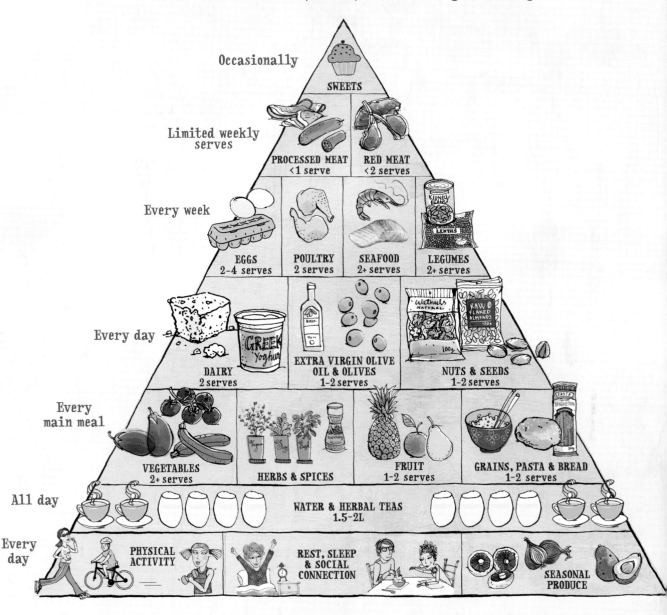

Occasionally

SWEETS

Limited weekly serves

PROCESSED MEAT
< 1 serve

RED MEAT
< 2 serves

Every week

EGGS
2-4 serves

POULTRY
2 serves

SEAFOOD
2+ serves

LEGUMES
2+ serves

Every day

DAIRY
2 serves

EXTRA VIRGIN OLIVE OIL & OLIVES
1-2 serves

NUTS & SEEDS
1-2 serves

Every main meal

VEGETABLES
2+ serves

HERBS & SPICES

FRUIT
1-2 serves

GRAINS, PASTA & BREAD
1-2 serves

All day

WATER & HERBAL TEAS
1.5-2L

Every day

PHYSICAL ACTIVITY

REST, SLEEP & SOCIAL CONNECTION

SEASONAL PRODUCE

HOW IT WORKS

At the top of the pyramid are the foods least associated with the Mediterranean diet eating pattern. As you go down the pyramid, layer by layer, the serving frequency increases with ingredients to incorporate into your life every day and even at every meal. At the base of the pyramid is the essence of the Mediterranean diet's way of living: physical activity, rest, sleep and social connection. Finally, there's the fundamental approach of eating what's in season for maximum freshness and nutrition.

It is also important to note that these serving sizes are only a guide, based on a healthy adult's needs. However, individuals have unique energy and nutrient requirements. For example, children, older adults, pregnant women and those with specific health conditions should adjust accordingly.

HOW MUCH IS A SERVE?

Occasionally

SWEETS
Opt for homemade versions based on wholegrains and fruit where possible

Limited weekly serves

PROCESSED MEAT
Serves: less than 1 per week
Includes salami, bacon, chorizo and sausages

RED MEAT
Serves: less than 2 per week
Choose lean cuts
• 1 serve = 90-100g raw or 65g cooked

Every week

EGGS
Serves: 2-4 per week
• 1 serve = 2 large eggs

POULTRY
Serves: 2 per week
• 1 serve = 80g cooked or 100g raw (lean)

SEAFOOD
Serves: 2 or more per week
Prioritise oily fish, such as sardines, mackerel and salmon
• 1 serve = 115g raw or 95g canned

LEGUMES
Serves: 2 or more per week
• 1 serve = 75g (½ cup cooked or canned)

Tofu
• 1 serve = 170g

Every day

DAIRY
Serves: 2 per day

Feta
• 1 serve = approx 40g (size of a matchbox)

Greek-style yoghurt
• 1 serve = 200g (¾ cup)

Low-fat milk
• 1 serve = 250ml (1 cup)

EXTRA VIRGIN OLIVE OIL & OLIVES
Serves: 1-2 per day
• 1 serve = 7g (1½ tsp)

NUTS & SEEDS
Serves: 1-2 per day
• 1 serve = 30g

Every main meal

VEGETABLES
Serves: 2 or more approx 75g per meal

Hard vegetables
Includes carrot, zucchini, green beans, broccoli, eggplant, capsicum and peas
• 1 serve = ½ cup

Leafy greens
Includes spinach and rocket
• 1 serve = 1 cup

Potatoes
Includes sweet potatoes
• 1 serve = ½ medium

Tomatoes
• 1 serve = 1 medium

HERBS & SPICES
Use to add flavour to meals

FRUIT
Serves: 1-2 approx 150g per meal

Medium sized
Includes apples, pears, oranges and bananas
• 1 serve = 1 fruit

Small sized
Includes plums, kiwifruit, nectarines and mandarins
• 1 serve = 2 fruits

Berries & fruit salad
• 1 serve = 1 cup

GRAINS, PASTA & BREAD
Serves: 1-2 serves per meal

Bread
• 1 serve = 1 slice bread or ½ bread roll

Grains
• 1 serve = 75-120g (½ cup) cooked

Oats
• 1 serve = 25g (¼ cup) uncooked

All day

WATER & HERBAL TEAS
Consume all day
Aim for at least 1.5-2L per day to ensure adequate hydration

Every day

SEASONAL PRODUCE
Eat fresh foods in season for the maximum intake of nutrients

7 DAY MEAL PLAN

Put the Mediterranean diet pyramid into practice with this week-long menu. We've balanced out your Monday to Sunday with everything you need.

BREAKFAST	LUNCH	DINNER

mon

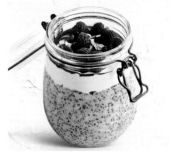
Nut Butter & Chia Overnight Oats **p38**

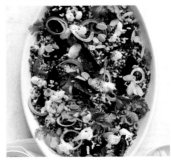
Warm Balsamic Beets & Lentils **p130**

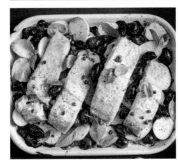
Speedy Olive & Salmon Bake **p214**

tues

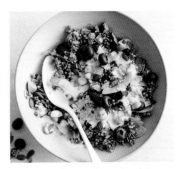
Cinnamon Ginger Granola **p34**

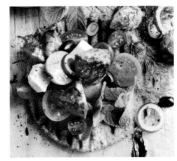
Greek Salad Chicken Pita **p52**

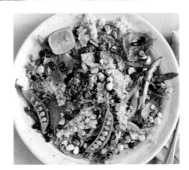
Super Green Quinoa Pilaf **p166**

wed

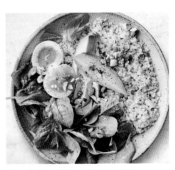
Egg & Avo Quinoa Bowl **p28**

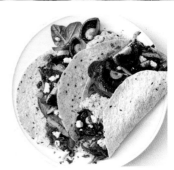
Mushroom & Capsicum Wraps **p66**

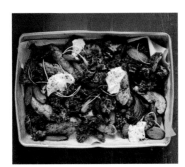
Harissa Chicken Tray Bake **p188**

	BREAKFAST	**LUNCH**	**DINNER**

thurs

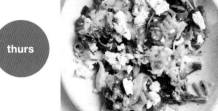

Vegie & Feta Scrambled Eggs **p40**

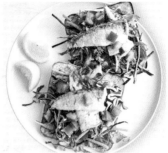

Kale Slaw Sardine Toasts **p90**

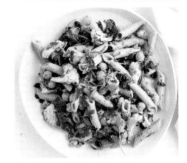

Buckwheat & Roast Cauli Pasta **p172**

fri

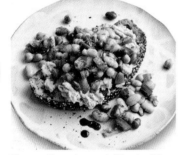

Tuscan Bean Avocado Toast **p32**

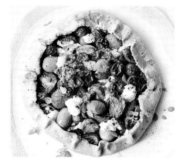

Tomato & Ricotta Spelt Tart **p62**

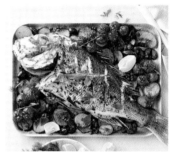

Potato & Snapper Bake **p168**

sat

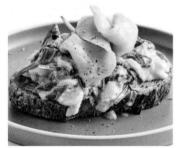

Salmon with Green Eggs **p26**

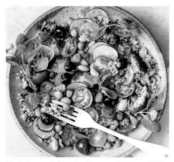

Rainbow & Fruity Power Plate **p126**

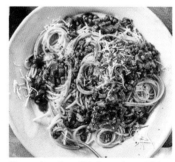

Gremolata Lentil Bolognaise **p186**

sun

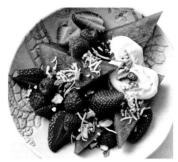

Quinoa & Red Fruit Salad **p44**

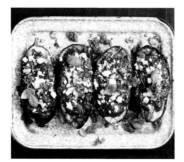

Greek Baked Eggplant **p80**

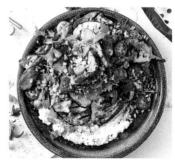

Freekeh & Cumin Lamb **p212**

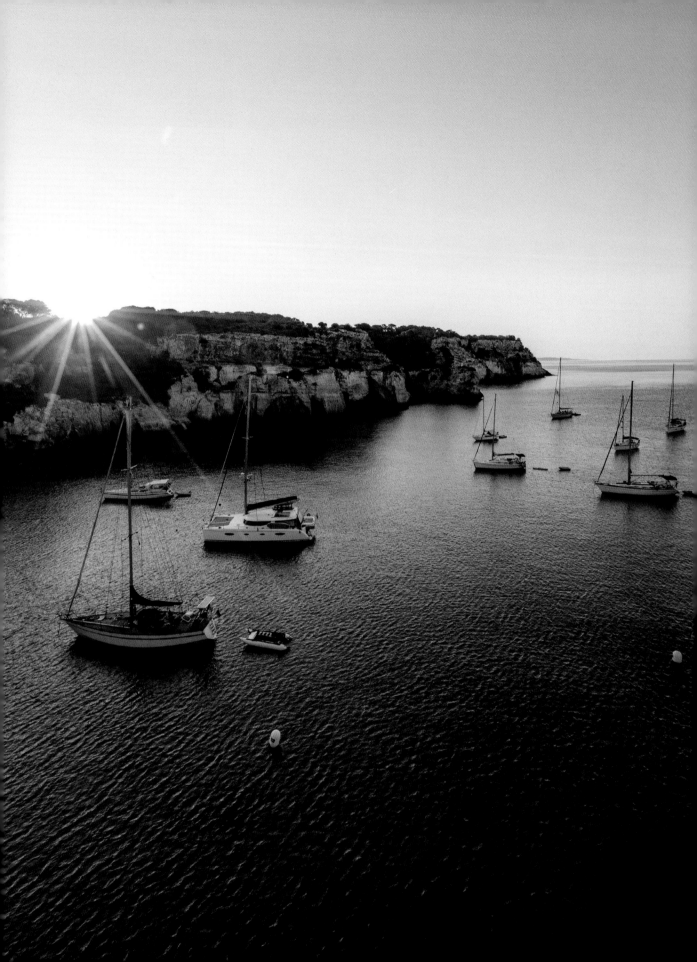

BREAKFAST

START YOUR DAY THE MEDITERRANEAN WAY WITH
WHOLEGRAINS, A RAINBOW OF FRUIT AND VEG,
AND A BIG HELPING OF NUTRIENTS!

Savoury FRENCH TOAST

Make your cooked breakfast a quick and vegie-loaded dish with our savoury twist on the weekend classic – ready in just 20 minutes.

SERVES 4 **PREP** 10 mins **COOK** 10 mins

250g cocktail truss tomatoes
4 eggs
80ml (⅓ cup) milk
8 slices wholemeal sourdough bread
1 small avocado, sliced
½ cup fresh basil leaves

1 Preheat oven to 180°C/160°C fan forced. Line a baking tray with baking paper.
2 Place the tomatoes on prepared tray and roast for 10 minutes or until slightly softened.
3 Whisk together the eggs and milk in a large shallow bowl.
4 Lightly spray a large non-stick frying pan with extra virgin olive oil and heat over medium heat. Dip 2 bread slices, 1 at a time, in the egg mixture until well soaked. Cook for 2 minutes each side or until golden and the egg is set. Repeat with the remaining bread and egg mixture.
5 Divide the French toast between serving plates. Top with the avocado, roasted tomatoes and basil. Season and serve.

COOK'S NOTE

Change up the toppings with your favourite in-season vegies and fresh herbs, such as mushrooms, kale and oregano.

NUTRITION (PER SERVE)

CALS	FAT	SAT FAT	PROTEIN	CARBS
253	15g	4g	12g	15g

★★★★★
Very tasty. Will definitely do again.
JANINE

● EASY ● QUICK ○ MAKE AHEAD ● MEAT FREE ● FAMILY FRIENDLY

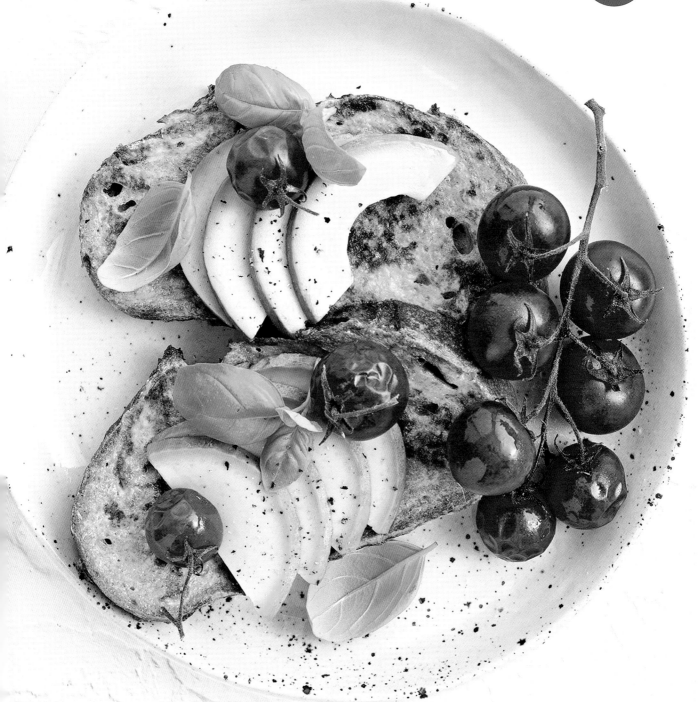

Almond & Blueberry
QUINOA SALAD

Quinoa for breakfast is a game-changer. It's a source of complete muscle-building protein and fibre. Blueberries add an antioxidant boost.

SERVES 4 **PREP** 10 mins (+ cooling) **COOK** 15 mins

135g (⅔ cup) quinoa, rinsed, drained
2 navel oranges
½ tsp ground cinnamon,
   plus extra to serve
2 tbs pepitas
2 tbs natural almonds, chopped
125g fresh blueberries
180g (⅔ cup) Greek-style yoghurt
   (optional)

1 Place the quinoa and 330ml (1⅓ cups) water in a saucepan over medium-high heat. Bring to the boil. Reduce heat to low and simmer, covered, for 12 minutes or until the water has evaporated and the quinoa is just tender. Transfer to a large bowl and set aside to cool.
2 Meanwhile, peel and segment the oranges over a bowl, reserving the juice.
3 Add the orange segments, reserved juice, cinnamon, pepitas, almonds and half the blueberries to the cooked quinoa. Stir until combined.
4 Divide the quinoa salad among serving bowls. Top with the remaining blueberries. Dollop with the yoghurt, if using. Sprinkle with extra cinnamon to serve.

COOK'S NOTE

For a nut-free version, replace the nuts with flaxseeds and sunflower seeds. The quinoa can be cooked up to 3 days in advance. Store in an airtight container in the fridge.

NUTRITION (PER SERVE)

CALS	FAT	SAT FAT	PROTEIN	CARBS
232	7g	1g	8g	31g

● EASY ● QUICK ● MAKE AHEAD ● MEAT FREE ● FAMILY FRIENDLY

★★★★★

Love this breakfast recipe! I usually eat mine at 8am and I'm never hungry before midday.

ALYSE-GRACE

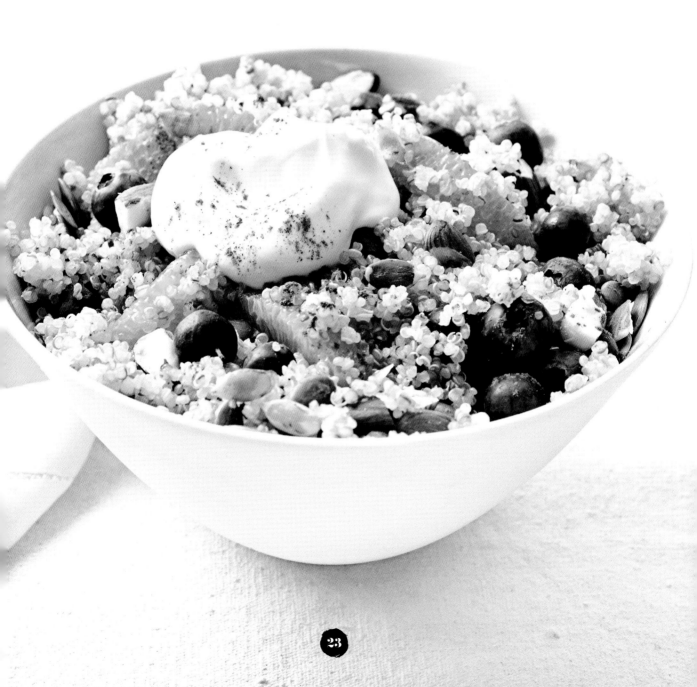

Watermelon & Berry
BUCKWHEAT

Everyone knows berries are a superfood, but don't forget watermelon. It's rich in vitamin C and potassium. Serve it with a simple, nutty granola.

SERVES 4 **PREP** 10 mins **COOK** 5 mins

2 tbs buckwheat, rinsed, drained, dried
2 tbs shredded coconut
2 tbs pistachio kernels, coarsely chopped
800g seedless watermelon, skin removed, cut into wedges
250g fresh strawberries, hulled, halved
125g fresh raspberries
180g (⅔ cup) Greek-style yoghurt

1 Preheat oven to 180°C/160°C fan forced. Line a baking tray with baking paper.
2 Combine the buckwheat, coconut and pistachio in a bowl. Spread the mixture over prepared tray and bake, stirring once, for 5 minutes or until light golden.
3 Arrange the watermelon, strawberry and raspberries on serving plates. Divide the buckwheat mixture among plates and top with the yoghurt.

COOK'S NOTE

Buckwheat is available in the health food aisle of the supermarket. Make sure you choose raw, not toasted.

NUTRITION (PER SERVE)

CALS	FAT	SAT FAT	PROTEIN	CARBS
188	7g	4g	7g	22g

★ ★ ★ ★ ★

Yum, I'll get out of bed for this combination of fresh fruit. Plus, I'm now sprinkling the granola on every sweet treat – so good!

FANCY FOODIE

● EASY ● QUICK ○ MAKE AHEAD ● MEAT FREE ● FAMILY FRIENDLY

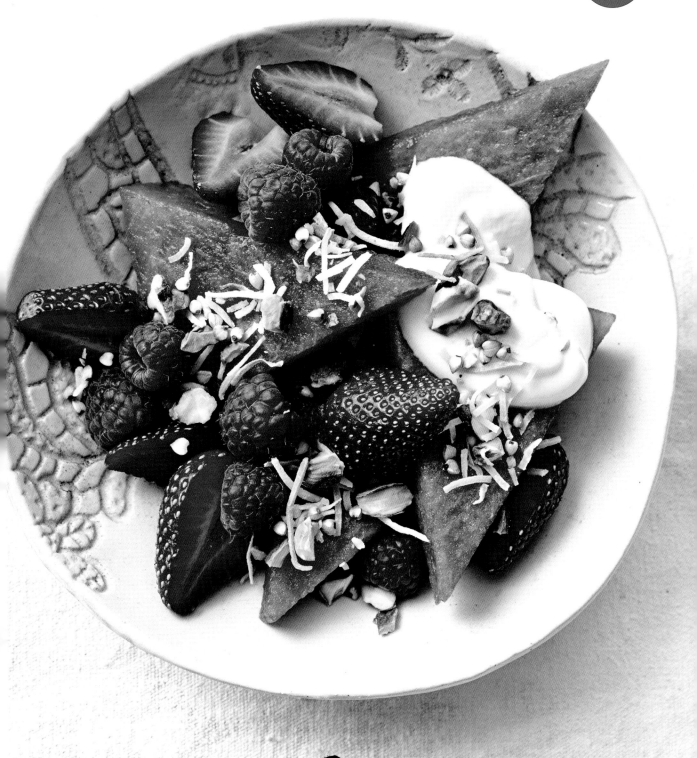

Salmon with
GREEN EGGS

For a protein-packed plate, top your toast with smoked salmon. It's also full of nutrients, vitamins and omega-3 fatty acids.

SERVES 4 **PREP** 5 mins **COOK** 5 mins

8 eggs
80 (⅓ cup) skim milk
120g baby spinach, coarsely
    chopped
4 slices wholegrain sourdough
    bread, toasted
100g smoked salmon slices

1 Whisk together the eggs and milk until well combined. Season.
2 Heat a non-stick frying pan over medium heat. Lightly spray with extra virgin olive oil. Add the spinach and cook, stirring, for 1 minute or until just wilted. Add the egg mixture and cook, folding gently with a wooden spatula, for 2-3 minutes or until the eggs are just set.
3 Top the toast with the egg mixture and salmon. Season with pepper to serve.

COOK'S NOTE

The secret to light and fluffy scrambled eggs is to whisk them well with milk before cooking.

NUTRITION (PER SERVE)

CALS	FAT	SAT FAT	PROTEIN	CARBS
323	17.1g	3.7g	24.6g	16.3g

★★★★★

Any excuse to eat smoked salmon and I'm in!
I've usually got these five ingredients on hand too.

FOODSLED

● EASY ● QUICK ○ MAKE AHEAD ○ MEAT FREE ○ FAMILY FRIENDLY

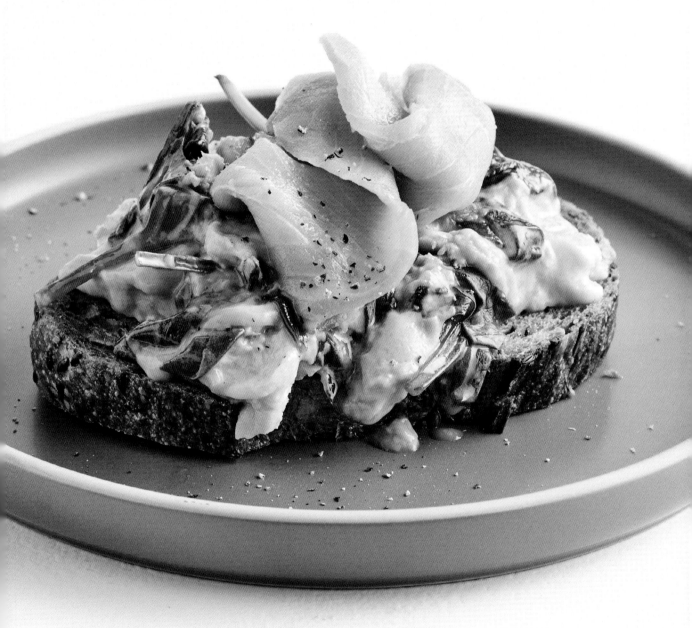

5
minutes
prep

Egg & Avo
QUINOA BOWL

Ready in just 10 minutes, this super veg bowl is full of quinoa, avocado and egg, so you're off to a great start.

SERVES 4 **PREP** 5 mins **COOK** 5 mins

4 eggs
300g (2 cups) cooked quinoa, warmed (see note)
200g baby spinach
1 avocado, sliced
1 tbs fresh lemon juice
1 tbs extra virgin olive oil
2 tbs chopped roasted unsalted almonds

1 Place the eggs in a small saucepan and cover with cold water from the tap. Bring to a gentle simmer over medium heat. Stir the water gently for 3 minutes for soft-boiled consistency. Use a slotted spoon to transfer the eggs to a chopping board. Carefully peel and halve.
2 Divide the quinoa, spinach, soft-boiled eggs and avocado among serving bowls. Drizzle over the lemon juice and oil.
3 Top with the almonds and season to serve.

COOK'S NOTE

To make 300g (2 cups) cooked quinoa, use about 100g uncooked.

NUTRITION (PER SERVE)

CALS	FAT	SAT FAT	PROTEIN	CARBS
277	18.2g	3g	11.4g	13.7g

Thank you for this recipe. It is wonderful to sit down on a weekend morning and slowly enjoy spoonfuls of quinoa and avo dripping in runny egg. Love it. **SHAWNTHEPRAWN**

● EASY   ● QUICK   ○ MAKE AHEAD   ● MEAT FREE   ● FAMILY FRIENDLY

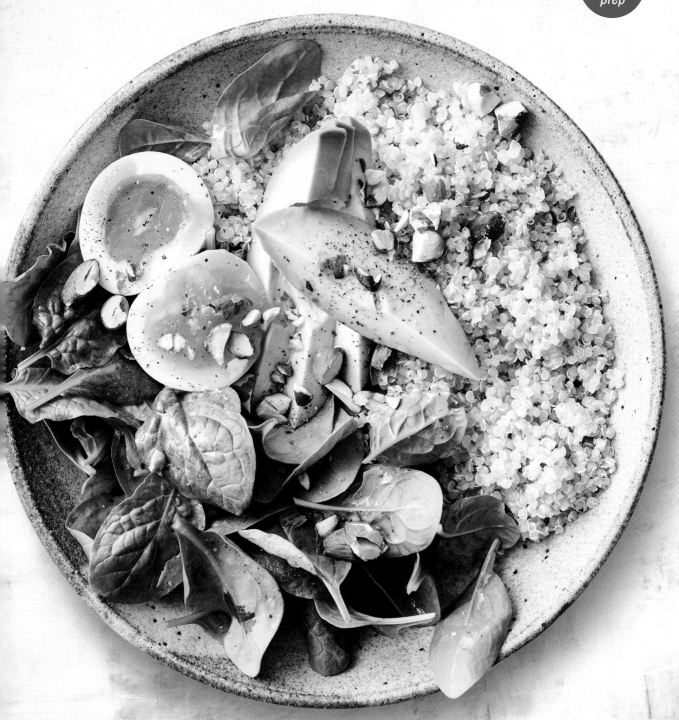

Strawberry & White Bean
PANCAKES

Fancy a pancake but don't want to break your diet? Try these lean white bean pancakes, topped with fresh fruit and honey.

SERVES 4 **PREP** 15 mins (+ 10 mins resting) **COOK** 15 mins

400g can cannellini beans, rinsed, drained

2 eggs

½ tsp vanilla extract

2 tbs honey

150g (1 cup) wholemeal self-raising flour

185ml (¾ cup) reduced-fat milk

150g fresh strawberries, hulled, sliced

Pulp of 2 passionfruit

1 Place the beans in a food processor and process until smooth. Add the eggs, vanilla and 1 tbs honey. Process until well combined. Transfer to a large bowl.

2 Sift over the flour. Pour in the milk and whisk until smooth. Set aside for 10 minutes to rest.

3 Heat a large non-stick frying pan over medium-high heat. Lightly spray with extra virgin olive oil. Ladle two ¼ cupfuls of the mixture into the pan. Cook for 3 minutes or until bubbles appear on the surface. Flip and cook for a further 1 minute or until light golden. Transfer to a plate and cover to keep warm. Repeat with the remaining mixture to make 8 pancakes in total.

4 Divide the pancakes among serving plates. Top with the strawberry and passionfruit pulp. Drizzle over the remaining honey to serve.

COOK'S NOTE

Top with any fresh fruit that's in season or omit the honey and make a savoury version topped with chopped tomato and avo.

NUTRITION (PER SERVE)

CALS	FAT	SAT FAT	PROTEIN	CARBS
298	5g	2g	13g	44g

● EASY ○ QUICK ○ MAKE AHEAD ● MEAT FREE ● FAMILY FRIENDLY

15+
minutes
prep

★★★★★

Simple and easy recipe and tastes fantastic. Happy to swap out any pancake recipe for this one now. Will remain in the favourites for sure!

GAROO

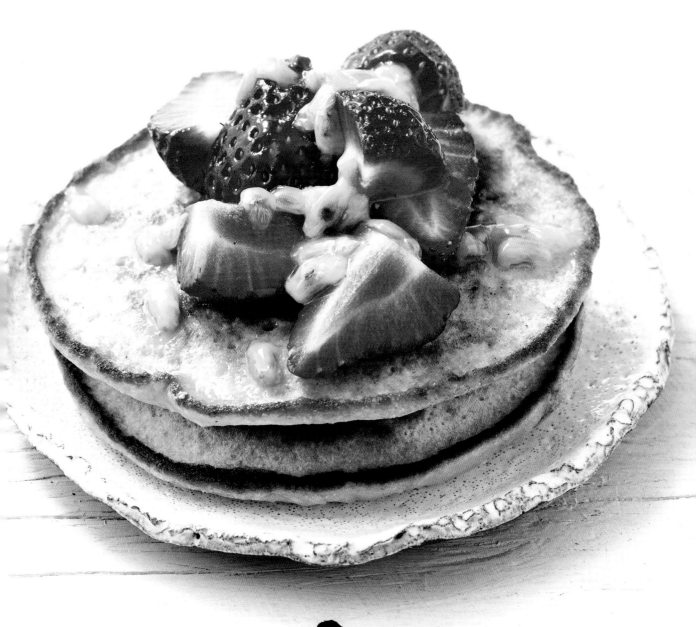

Tuscan Bean
AVOCADO TOAST

Mix canned beans and whatever veg you have to make this nourishing breakfast – also awesome as an afternoon pick-me-up or lazy dinner!

SERVES 4 **PREP** 5 mins

- 4 x 125g cans four bean mix, rinsed, drained
- 4 small vine-ripened tomatoes, finely chopped
- ⅓ cup chopped fresh continental parsley leaves
- 1 tbs balsamic vinegar
- 4 slices wholegrain sourdough bread, toasted
- 1 small avocado, mashed
- 1 tbs extra virgin olive oil

1 Combine the beans, tomato, parsley and vinegar in a bowl. Season.
2 Spread the toast with the avocado then top with the bean mixture. Drizzle over the oil, season and serve.

NUTRITION (PER SERVE)

CALS	FAT	SAT FAT	PROTEIN	CARBS
304	9.8g	1.5g	12.1g	35.6g

COOK'S NOTE

Replace the four bean mix with canned chickpeas, black beans or red kidney beans, if you prefer.

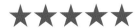

I always stay fuller for longer when I chow down on beans, so I love tucking into this toast for breakfast.

FRIDGETUNER

● EASY ● QUICK ○ MAKE AHEAD ● MEAT FREE ○ FAMILY FRIENDLY

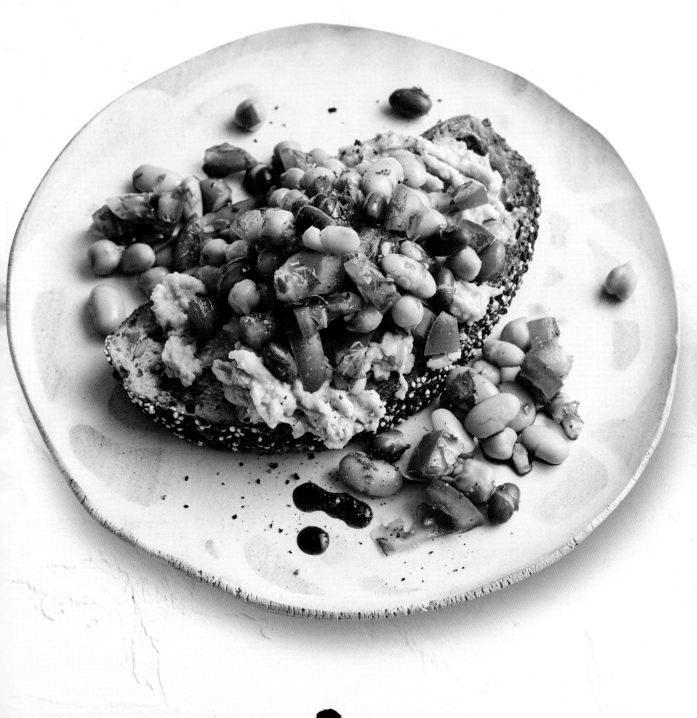

Cinnamon GINGER GRANOLA

These golden clusters use only natural sweeteners, but still have that crunch. It's a quick go-to option – just add yoghurt or milk.

MAKES 6 cups (½ cup per serve) **PREP** 15 mins (+ cooling) **COOK** 20 mins

2 tbs extra virgin olive oil
40g (2 cups) puffed quinoa
200g (1 cup) mixed chopped nuts
   (such as cashews, almonds,
   walnuts, brazil nuts)
90g (1 cup) rolled oats
30g (½ cup) coconut flakes
45g (¼ cup) pepitas
2 tbs chia seeds
2 tbs hemp seeds
2-3 tsp finely grated fresh ginger,
   to taste
1 vanilla bean, split
1½ tsp ground cinnamon
½ tsp ground cardamom
½ tsp ground cloves
1½ tbs honey
Greek-style yoghurt and fresh
   blueberries, to serve (optional)

1 Preheat oven to 180°C/160°C fan forced. Line 2 baking trays with baking paper.
2 Place the oil, puffed quinoa, mixed nuts, oats, coconut, pepitas, chia and hemp seeds, ginger, vanilla seeds, cinnamon, cardamom, cloves and 1 tbs honey in a large bowl. Stir until well coated.
3 Divide the mixture among prepared trays, spreading out evenly. Bake for 10 minutes. Stir with a spatula. Bake for a further 5-10 minutes or until light golden and crisp.
4 Drizzle over the remaining honey. Mix well. Set aside on the trays to cool completely.
5 Serve with yoghurt and blueberries, if using.

NUTRITION (PER SERVE)

CALS	FAT	SAT FAT	PROTEIN	CARBS
253	19.2g	5.8g	6.6g	12.2g

COOK'S NOTE

Puffed quinoa has a slightly nutty taste and crispiness. Find at health food stores and some delis. Store the granola in an airtight container in a cool, dry place for up to 2 weeks.

★★★★★

My 15 year old daughter made this. The flavour was amazing. Definitely don't need the sweetness many commercial varieties put in. Great healthy start for the day. **ROSEPYLE**

● EASY   ○ QUICK   ● MAKE AHEAD   ● MEAT FREE   ● FAMILY FRIENDLY

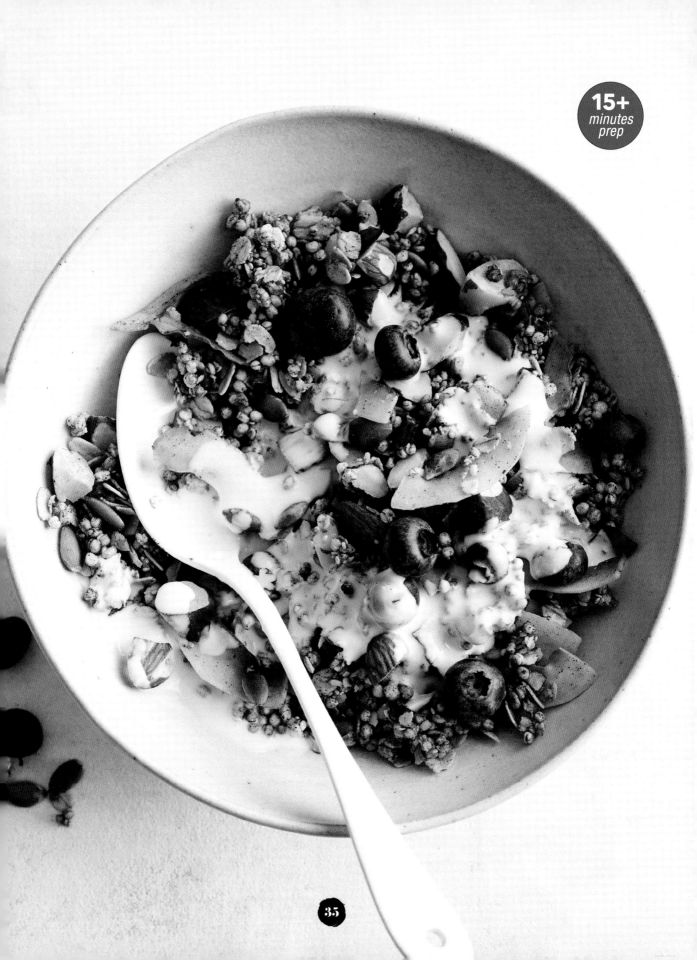

Baked Egg & Kale
HERB POTS

Eggs are a staple of the Mediterranean diet for good reason – they're loaded with essential vitamins and minerals, antioxidants and omega-3 fatty acids.

SERVES 4 **PREP** 15 mins (+ cooling) **COOK** 30 mins

2 tsp extra virgin olive oil

250g peeled sweet potato, coarsely grated

80g trimmed kale leaves, chopped

2 garlic cloves, crushed

8 eggs

60g Greek feta, crumbled

⅔ cup chopped fresh herb leaves (such as parsley and basil)

100g chargrilled red capsicum (not in oil), thinly sliced

2 tsp fresh lemon juice

1 Preheat oven to 180°C/160°C fan forced. Lightly spray four 350ml ovenproof ramekins with oil.

2 Heat the oil in a large frying pan over medium-high heat. Cook the sweet potato, stirring, for 3-4 minutes or until softened. Add the kale and garlic. Cook, stirring, for 2 minutes or until wilted. Set aside to cool slightly.

3 Whisk the eggs in a bowl. Stir in the feta, most of the herbs and sweet potato mixture. Ladle the mixture into prepared ramekins and bake for 25 minutes or until puffed, golden and set.

4 Combine the capsicum, lemon juice and remaining herbs in a small bowl. Serve pots topped with capsicum mixture.

COOK'S NOTE

Don't have sweet potato and kale on hand? Try grated carrot, zucchini or potato, and spinach or rocket.

NUTRITION (PER SERVE)

CALS	FAT	SAT FAT	PROTEIN	CARBS
271	16g	5g	18g	11g

★★★★★

Wow, this is delicious! Very moreish, I normally don't make these sort of dishes as I find the taste too eggy. This is not the case here!

C1CD

● EASY ○ QUICK ○ MAKE AHEAD ● MEAT FREE ● FAMILY FRIENDLY

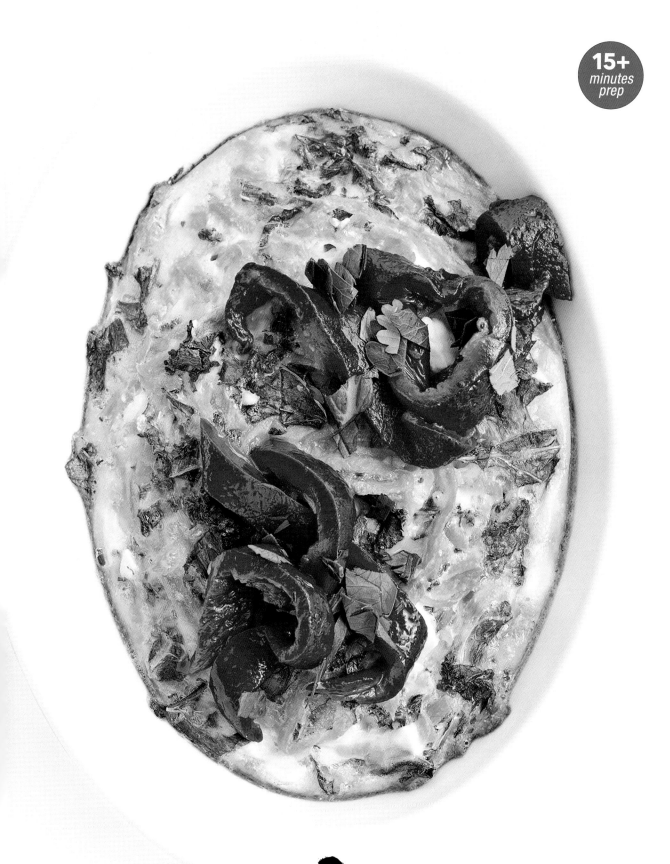

Nut Butter & Chia
OVERNIGHT OATS

When you've got a busy morning and are basically flying out the door,
you'll be thankful you prepared this mighty jar the night before!

SERVES 4 **PREP** 5 mins (+ overnight soaking)

120g (1⅓ cups) rolled oats
2 tbs chia seeds
2 tbs pepitas, plus extra to serve
1 tbs nut butter (such as almond or natural peanut butter)
1 tsp ground cinnamon
500ml (2 cups) unsweetened almond or skim milk
1 tbs honey
180g (⅔ cup) Greek-style yoghurt
160g (1⅓ cups) fresh or frozen raspberries

1 Combine the oats, chia seeds, pepitas, nut butter, cinnamon, milk and honey in 4 airtight jars or containers. Cover and place in the fridge overnight to soak.
2 Top the oat mixture with the yoghurt, raspberries and extra pepitas to serve.

NUTRITION (PER SERVE)

CALS	FAT	SAT FAT	PROTEIN	CARBS
279	12.9g	2.9g	10.3g	26g

COOK'S NOTE

This is great to feed a family of four for brekky or a couple over 2 days as the overnight oats will keep in the fridge for 2 days.

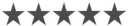

These taste great and are super easy to make. Followed the recipe exactly. **LG22**

● EASY ○ QUICK ● MAKE AHEAD ● MEAT FREE ● FAMILY FRIENDLY

5+
*minutes
prep*

★★★★★

Perfect amount. Keeps you full without feeling bloated.
MCHARLIE

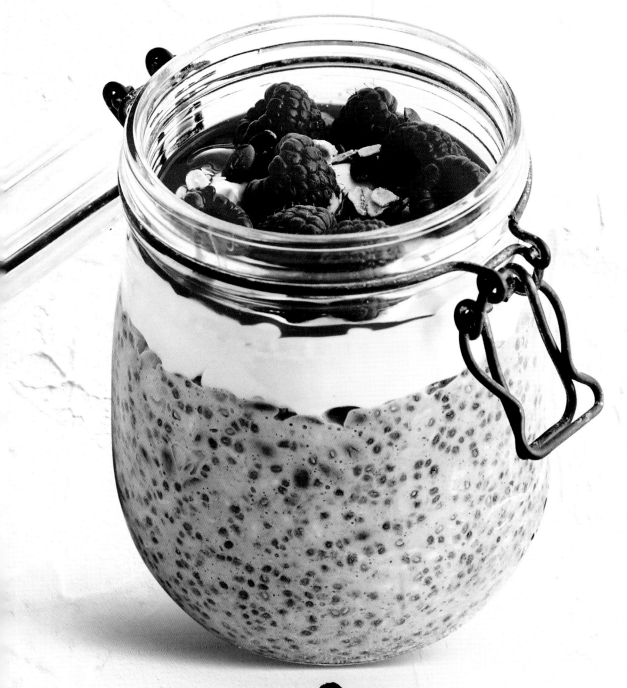

Vegie & Feta
SCRAMBLED EGGS

Pack your scrambie eggs with veg that'll boost the flavour and your intake of goodness with this fry-up – ready in just 15 minutes!

SERVES 4 **PREP** 5 mins **COOK** 10 mins

1 tbs extra virgin olive oil

300g sweet potato, peeled, coarsely grated

4 small vine-ripened tomatoes, finely chopped

8 green shallots, thinly sliced

8 eggs, lightly whisked

80g baby spinach

80g Greek feta, crumbled

1 Heat the oil in a non-stick frying pan over medium-high heat. Add the sweet potato, tomato and shallot. Cook, stirring, for 3 minutes or until softened. Season.

2 Reduce heat to low. Add the egg and cook, gently folding the egg with a wooden spatula, for 3-4 minutes or until just set. Add the spinach and fold through until just wilted. Sprinkle with the feta and season. Divide among serving plates.

COOK'S NOTE

If you want to serve this with toast, choose a wholegrain sourdough bread.

NUTRITION (PER SERVE)

CALS	FAT	SAT FAT	PROTEIN	CARBS
295	16.9g	5.3g	18.5g	15.1g

★★★★★

Who knew you could jam so much good stuff into scrambled eggs and it still tastes great?! This is a winner.

WAFFLEISO

● EASY ● QUICK ○ MAKE AHEAD ● MEAT FREE ● FAMILY FRIENDLY

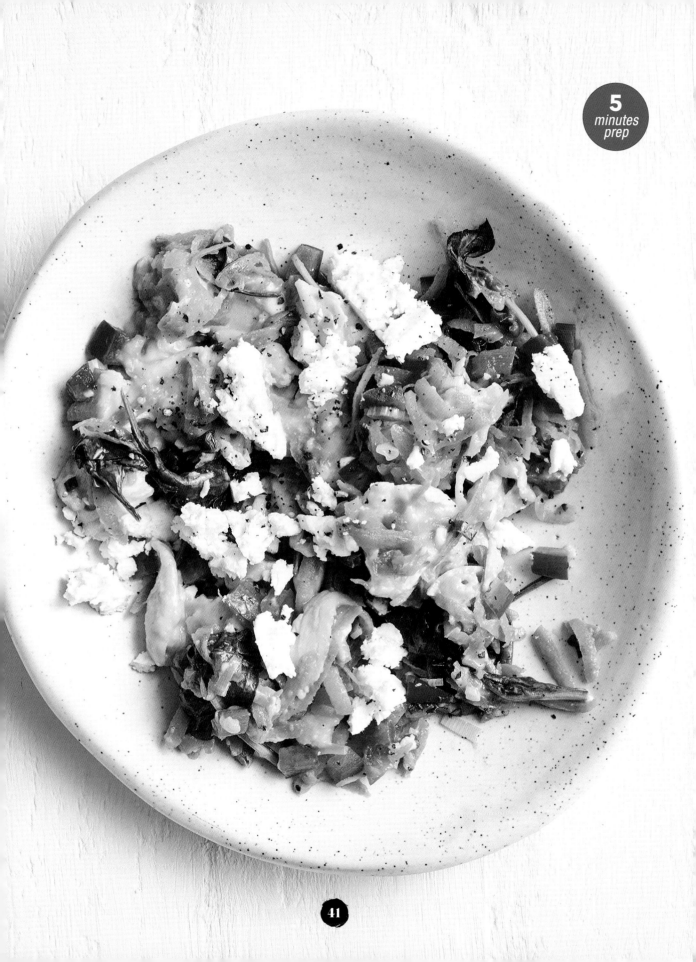

5
minutes
prep

Avo & Chilli
BLACK BEAN WRAP

This wholesome wrap is as easy as mashing black beans
with lemon and chilli, and topping with fresh vegies.

SERVES 4 **PREP** 10 mins

4 x 125g cans black beans,
  rinsed, drained
Large pinch of dried chilli flakes
2 tbs fresh lemon juice
4 wholegrain wraps
80g baby spinach
4 roma tomatoes, sliced
1 avocado, sliced
⅔ cup fresh basil leaves
Lemon wedges, to serve (optional)

1 Coarsely mash the black beans in a bowl. Stir in the
chilli and lemon juice. Season.
2 Spread the bean mixture over each wrap. Arrange
the spinach, tomato, avocado and basil on top.
Serve with lemon wedges to squeeze over, if using.

NUTRITION (PER SERVE)

CALS	FAT	SAT FAT	PROTEIN	CARBS
285	8.7g	1.9g	11.3g	32.2g

**COOK'S
NOTE**

If you prefer your
wrap toasted,
fold over the filled
wrap to enclose
then toast in a
sandwich press
until golden
and crisp.

★★★★★

*I would never have thought of mashed black beans as being
a tasty filling, but they really hit the spot. Super easy too.*
HARMONYPUFFIN

● EASY ● QUICK ○ MAKE AHEAD ● MEAT FREE ○ FAMILY FRIENDLY

10
minutes
prep

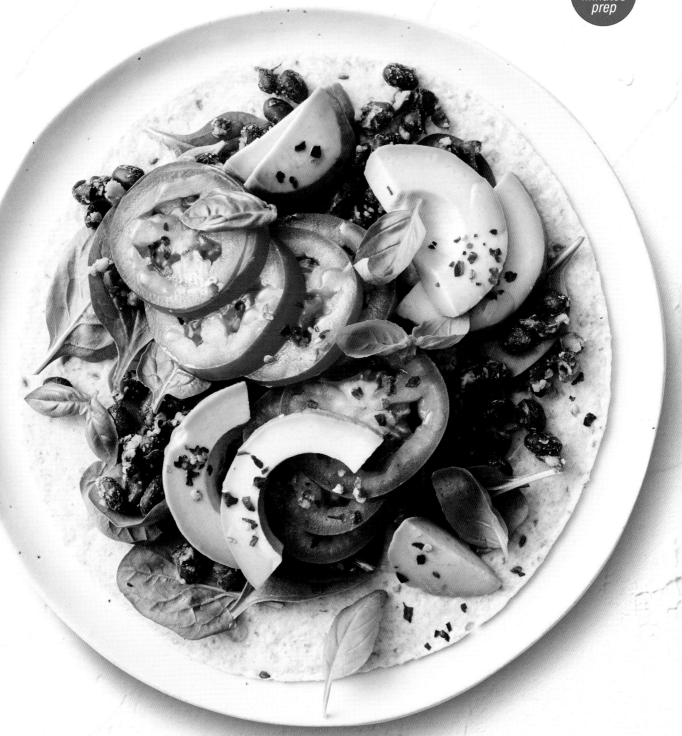

Quinoa & Red
FRUIT SALAD

Avoid the morning rush by prepping this beautiful brekky bowl the night before. Added bonus: it's full of heart-healthy ingredients.

SERVES 4 **PREP** 15 mins **COOK** 15 mins

100g (½ cup) tri-colour quinoa, rinsed, drained
2 passionfruit, halved
1 tbs fresh lime juice
500g piece watermelon, peeled, very thinly sliced
250g fresh strawberries, hulled, quartered
125g fresh raspberries
150g fresh cherries, pitted, halved
1 Jazz apple, thinly sliced crossways
2 tbs finely shredded fresh mint leaves

1 Cook the quinoa in a saucepan following packet directions. Drain and refresh under cold running water.
2 Scoop out the passionfruit pulp and place in a jug with the lime juice. Stir until combined.
3 Divide the watermelon, strawberry, raspberries, cherry and apple among serving plates. Top with the quinoa then drizzle over the passionfruit mixture. Sprinkle with the mint to serve

NUTRITION (PER SERVE)

CALS	FAT	SAT FAT	PROTEIN	CARBS
179	1.9g	0.2g	5g	29.9g

COOK'S NOTE

The quinoa can be cooked up to 3 days in advance. Store in an airtight container in the fridge.

★★★★★

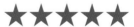

This is such a good idea to make fruit salad substantial – it sustains me through until lunch.

BAKINGSELFIES

● EASY ● QUICK ● MAKE AHEAD ● MEAT FREE ● FAMILY FRIENDLY

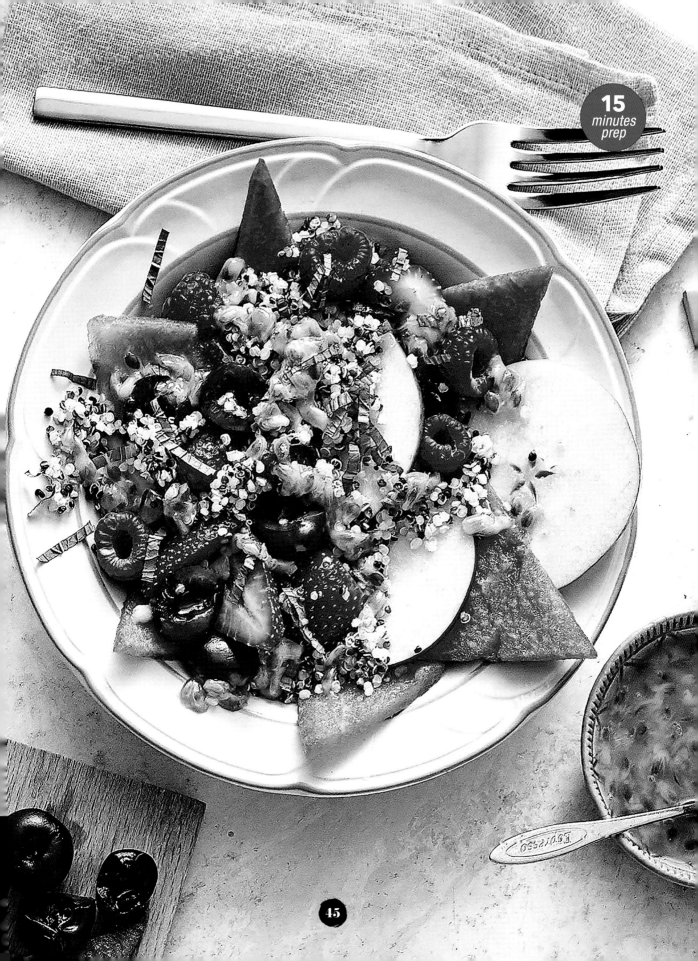

15 minutes prep

45

Smashed Chickpea
BRUSCHETTA

This legume smash is the toast with the most! We're talking protein, fibre and healthy fats that can help you manage cholesterol and blood pressure.

SERVES 4 **PREP** 5 mins

4 x 125g cans chickpeas, rinsed, drained
1 tbs fresh lemon juice
1 tbs tahini
200g cherry tomatoes, quartered
⅓ cup chopped fresh continental parsley leaves
2 tsp extra virgin olive oil
4 slices wholegrain bread, toasted
Lemon wedges, to serve

1 Place the chickpeas, lemon juice and tahini in a small bowl. Mash with a fork, leaving some texture. Season.
2 Combine the tomato, parsley and oil in a small bowl. Spread the chickpea mixture over the toast. Top with the tomato salad. Serve with lemon wedges to squeeze over.

NUTRITION (PER SERVE)

CALS	FAT	SAT FAT	PROTEIN	CARBS
256	10g	1g	11g	25g

COOK'S NOTE

Make the mashed chickpea mixture up to 2 days ahead. In fact, you could double it to have on hand for another meal.

★★★★★

I actually really love this and have added it on my regular breakfast rotation. Easy, tasty and keeps me going. I add a small amount of garlic to the chickpea mix. **FRANGIPANIANGIE**

● EASY ● QUICK ● MAKE AHEAD ● MEAT FREE ● FAMILY FRIENDLY

★★★★★

We had this for Sunday breakfast. Great healthy alternative.

HBN

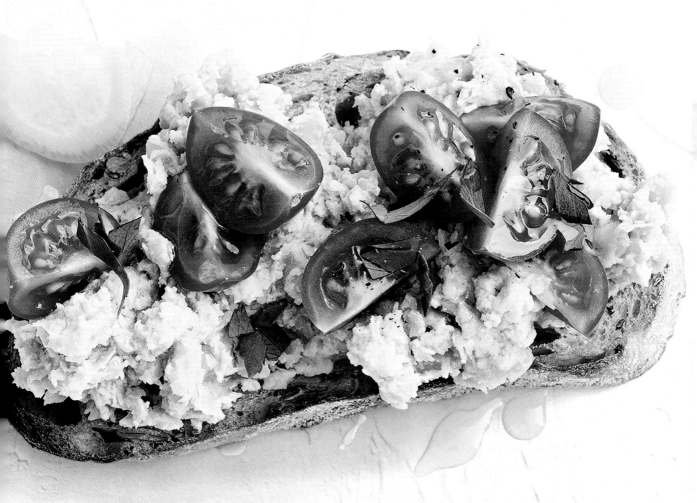

Spinach & Bean
SCRAMBLE

You only need six ingredients to whip up these
fresh and fast scrambled eggs – ready in just 10 minutes.

SERVES 4 **PREP** 5 mins **COOK** 5 mins

8 eggs
160ml (⅔ cup) unsweetened almond
  or skim milk
1 tbs extra virgin olive oil
4 x 125g cans black beans,
  rinsed, drained
120g baby spinach
80g Greek feta, crumbled

1 Whisk the eggs and milk in a small bowl. Season.
2 Heat a non-stick frying pan over medium heat then add
the oil. Cook the beans and spinach, stirring, for 1-2 minutes
or until spinach is wilted. Transfer to a bowl.
3 Pour the egg mixture into the pan and cook, gently folding
with a wooden spatula, until the egg is just set. Stir through
the bean mixture. Sprinkle with the feta and season to serve.

**COOK'S
NOTE**

This is also
delicious served
in a wholegrain
wrap with a dash
of chilli sauce as
a brekky burrito,
if you like.

NUTRITION (PER SERVE)

CALS	FAT	SAT FAT	PROTEIN	CARBS
280	15.4g	4.5g	20.7g	11.1g

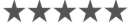

Was lovely... fresh and filling! I added chilli flakes to give it a kick!
BECRIDD

● EASY ● QUICK ○ MAKE AHEAD ● MEAT FREE ● FAMILY FRIENDLY

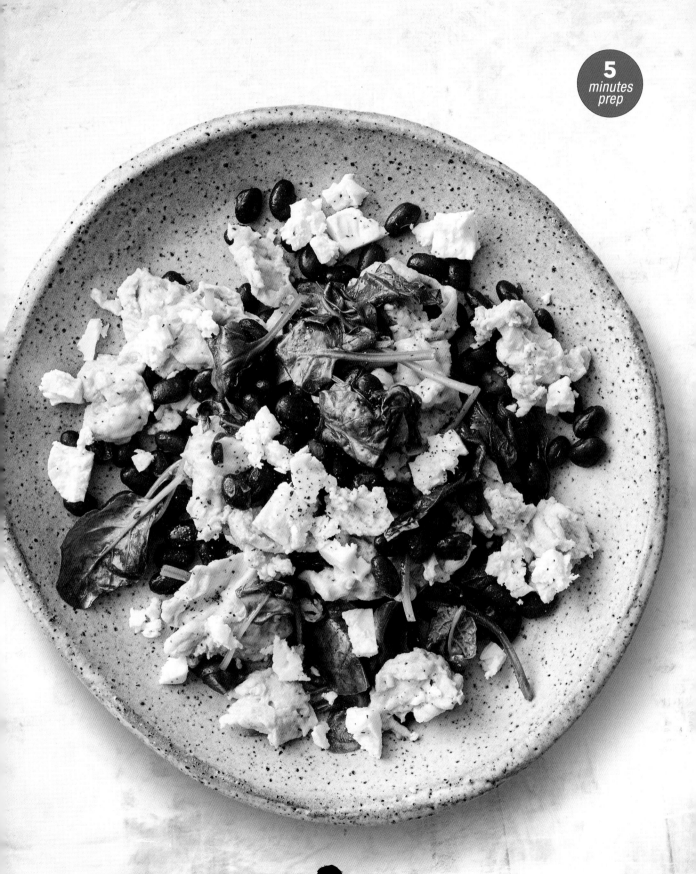

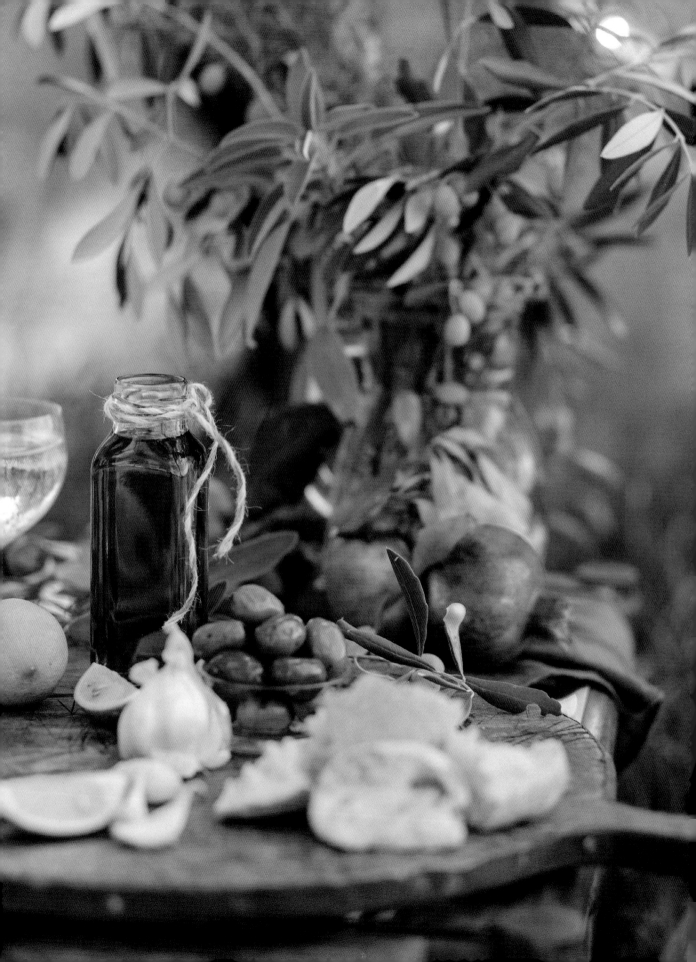

SMALL MEALS & SNACKS

THE 3PM SLUMP IS A RISKY TIME OF DAY FOR EATING WELL, BUT DON'T WORRY WE'VE GOT YOU COVERED WHEN THE HANGRIES HIT. WANT A LIGHT LUNCH? THEY'RE IN HERE TOO.

Greek Salad-Topped CHICKEN PITA

If there's a meal that screams flavours of the Med, this is it! The trick will be rolling the pita after you've loaded it with all the amazing fillings.

SERVES 6 **PREP** 30 mins (+ 1 hour marinating) **COOK** 10 mins

2 large garlic cloves, crushed
1 lemon, rind finely grated
1 tbs fresh lemon juice (see note)
60ml (¼ cup) extra virgin olive oil
2 large (about 750g) chicken breast
  fillets, cut into 2cm pieces
1 tbs balsamic vinegar
1 tbs honey
4 small wholemeal pita bread,
  chargrilled

TZATZIKI
1 Lebanese cucumber, peeled,
  coarsely grated
200g Greek-style yoghurt
1 large garlic clove, crushed
2 tsp fresh lemon juice
1 tbs fresh dill, chopped
1 tbs fresh mint leaves, chopped

GREEK SALAD
350g pkt tomato medley mix, halved
150g Greek feta, cut into cubes
100g kalamata olives, pitted
½ red onion, sliced into rings
¼ cup fresh dill
¼ cup fresh mint leaves
2 tbs extra virgin olive oil
2 tsp red wine vinegar

1 Combine the garlic, lemon rind, lemon juice and 2 tbs oil in a large bowl. Season. Add the chicken and toss to combine. Cover and place in the fridge for 1 hour to marinate.
2 Meanwhile, make the tzatziki. Squeeze the excess liquid from the cucumber. Pat dry with paper towel. Place in a bowl with the remaining tzatziki ingredients. Season. Stir to combine. Cover and place in the fridge until required.
3 To make the Greek salad, place the tomato, feta, olives, onion, dill and mint in a bowl. Combine the oil and red wine vinegar in a small bowl. Season. Add to the salad and toss to combine.
4 Heat half the remaining oil in a large non-stick frying pan over medium-high heat. Add half the marinated chicken and cook, turning, for 3-4 minutes or until golden and cooked through. Transfer to a plate. Repeat with the remaining oil and chicken. Return all the chicken to the pan. Add the balsamic vinegar and honey. Cook, stirring, for 1 minute or until caramelised.
5 Divide the chicken and Greek salad among the pita and serve with the tzatziki on the side.

COOK'S NOTE

Juice the lemon that you've grated the rind from (for the marinade). Marinate the chicken for up to 24 hours and make the tzatziki up to 24 hours ahead too.

NUTRITION (PER SERVE)

CALS	FAT	SAT FAT	PROTEIN	CARBS
458	21.9g	7.1g	37.4g	25g

○ EASY ○ QUICK ● MAKE AHEAD ○ MEAT FREE ● FAMILY FRIENDLY

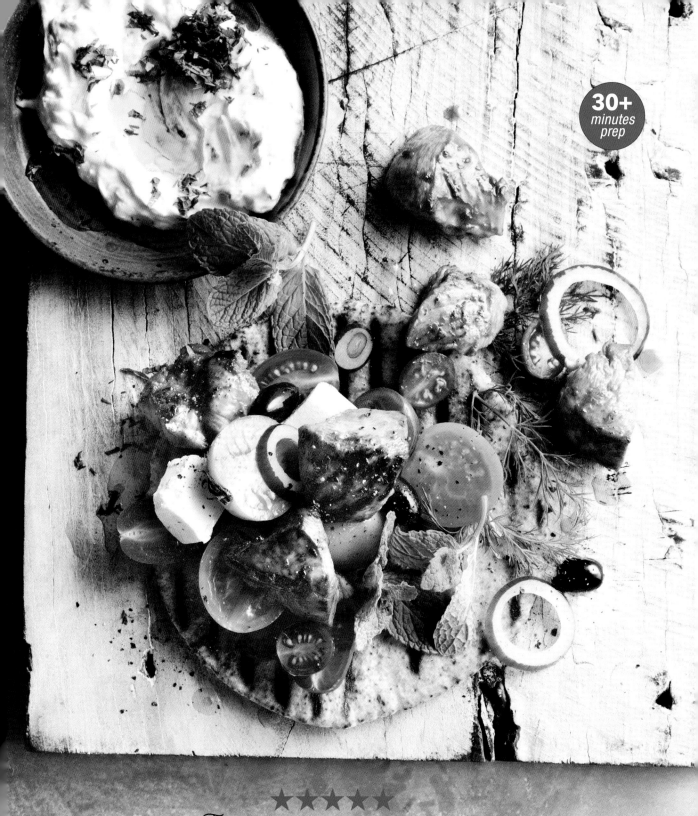

★★★★★

*This is a great summer dinner.
I'd definitely serve it for a casual dinner party too.*

ESMEWATSON

5-Minute Egg & Hummus
FLATBREAD

This super veg lunch is quick to throw together and will easily travel too. Just fill, roll and tie up with string or wrap in foil and you're ready to go.

SERVES 4 **PREP** 5 mins

90g (⅓ cup) hummus
4 wholegrain wraps
80g baby rocket
2 Lebanese cucumber, cut into matchsticks (see note)
200g cherry tomatoes, halved
40g Greek feta, crumbled
4 soft-boiled eggs, peeled, halved
⅓ cup chopped fresh continental parsley leaves

1 Spread the hummus over the wraps. Top with the rocket, cucumber, tomato, feta, egg and parsley. Season and serve.

NUTRITION (PER SERVE)

CALS	FAT	SAT FAT	PROTEIN	CARBS
289	13.8g	4.3g	14.5g	23.2g

COOK'S NOTE

If you have a spiraliser, use it to cut the cucumber into noodles to spread over the wrap.

★★★★★

Yum! Enjoyed this for my work lunch, then gave it a run in my teenager's lunchbox. It came home empty – winning!

VIOLAPARMESAN

● EASY ● QUICK ○ MAKE AHEAD ● MEAT FREE ● FAMILY FRIENDLY

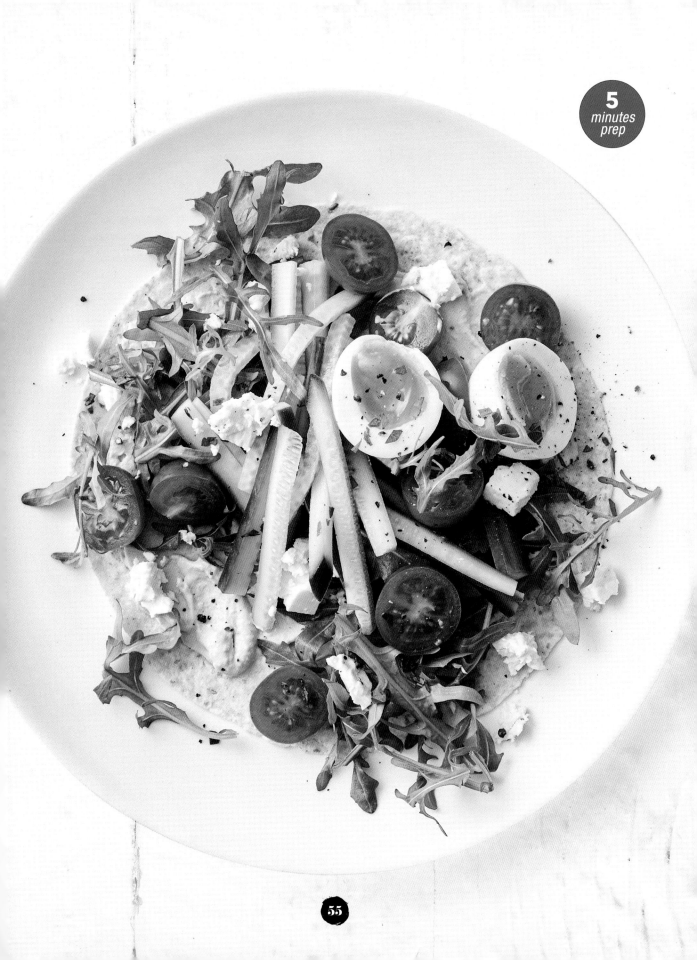

Healthy Pumpkin
ZUCCHINI SLICE

Take your zucchini slice game to the next level
by adding red onion, pumpkin, tomato, quinoa and feta.

SERVES 4 **PREP** 20 mins (+ cooling) **COOK** 40 mins

2 tsp extra virgin olive oil
1 red onion, finely chopped
2 garlic cloves, crushed
350g butternut pumpkin, peeled,
   deseeded, coarsely grated
2 zucchini, coarsely grated
8 eggs
150g (1 cup) cooked quinoa
60g Greek feta, crumbled
2 tbs chopped fresh basil leaves
250g cherry tomatoes, halved
80g baby rocket

1 Preheat oven to 190ºC/170ºC fan forced. Line a
16 x 26cm (base size) baking pan with baking paper.
2 Heat the oil in a large non-stick frying pan over high
heat. Add the onion and cook, stirring, for 3 minutes or
until softened. Add the garlic and cook, stirring, for 1 minute
or until aromatic. Add the pumpkin. Cook, stirring, for
2-3 minutes or until softened. Add the zucchini. Cook,
stirring, for 1-2 minutes or until bright green. Set aside
to cool slightly.
3 Whisk the eggs in a large bowl until combined. Stir in
the vegetable mixture, quinoa, feta and basil.
4 Pour the mixture into prepared pan. Top with half the
tomato, cut-side up. Bake for 25-30 minutes or until golden
and cooked through. Set aside to cool slightly before serving
with rocket and remaining tomato on top.

COOK'S NOTE

This slice will keep
in the fridge for
up to 3 days, so
keep any leftovers
to take to work
for lunch. Serve
with wholegrain
sourdough bread,
if you like.

NUTRITION (PER SERVE)

CALS	FAT	SAT FAT	PROTEIN	CARBS
303	16.3g	5.9g	20.4g	16.1g

★★★★★

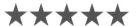

*I loved this one. Super easy and good to mix it up
if you don't have all the ingredients.* **STEPHLYPEPHLY**

● EASY ○ QUICK ● MAKE AHEAD ● MEAT FREE ● FAMILY FRIENDLY

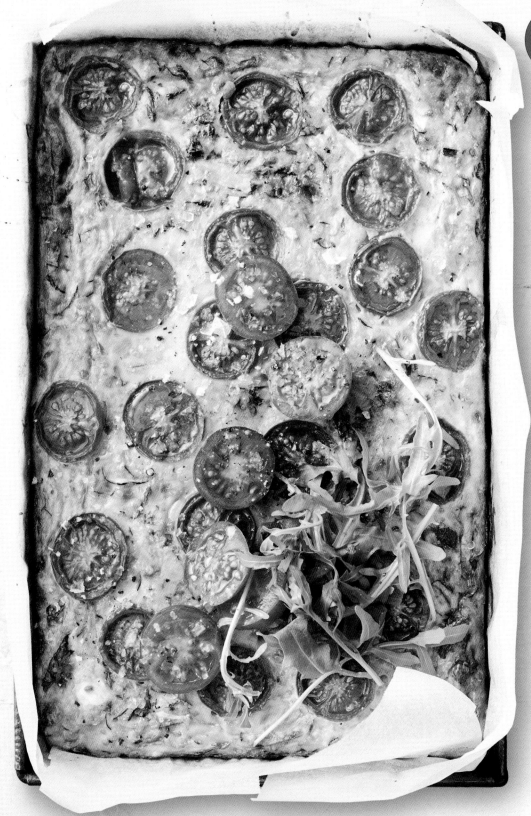

20+
minutes
prep

Prawn & Avo
PITA BITES

A twist on the classic prawn cocktail, these morsels are party worthy, but easy enough to make for a snack, especially with the make-ahead pita crisps.

MAKES 16 **PREP** 20 mins **COOK** 10 mins

1 wholemeal Lebanese bread
1 small avocado, halved
1 tbs fresh lemon juice
2 tbs hummus
16 medium peeled cooked
    prawns, deveined
3 radishes, cut into matchsticks
16 small watercress sprigs
Ground sumac, to serve

1 Preheat oven to 200°C/180°C fan forced. Line a large baking tray with baking paper.
2 Use scissors to trim the bread into a large rough square then cut into 16 small squares. Arrange in a single layer on prepared tray. Spray with extra virgin olive oil and season. Bake for 6 minutes or until golden and crisp. Set aside to cool.
3 Meanwhile, scoop the avocado into a bowl. Coarsely mash. Add half the lemon juice. Season and stir to combine. Place the hummus in a separate bowl. Add the remaining lemon juice. Stir to combine.
4 Spread each pita square with the avocado mixture then the hummus mixture. Arrange the bites on a serving platter or board. Top with the prawns, radish and watercress. Sprinkle with sumac.

COOK'S NOTE

Make the crispy pita squares up to 1 week ahead – and that includes the offcuts too! Once cool, store in an airtight container. They're also delicious on a cheeseboard or dip plate.

NUTRITION (EACH)

CALS	FAT	SAT FAT	PROTEIN	CARBS
43	2.2g	0.4g	1.9g	3.6g

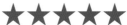

★★★★★

These were a great budget option for our drinks party. So easy, so fresh.
DANI.BROUGHAM

● EASY ● QUICK ● MAKE AHEAD ○ MEAT FREE ● FAMILY FRIENDLY

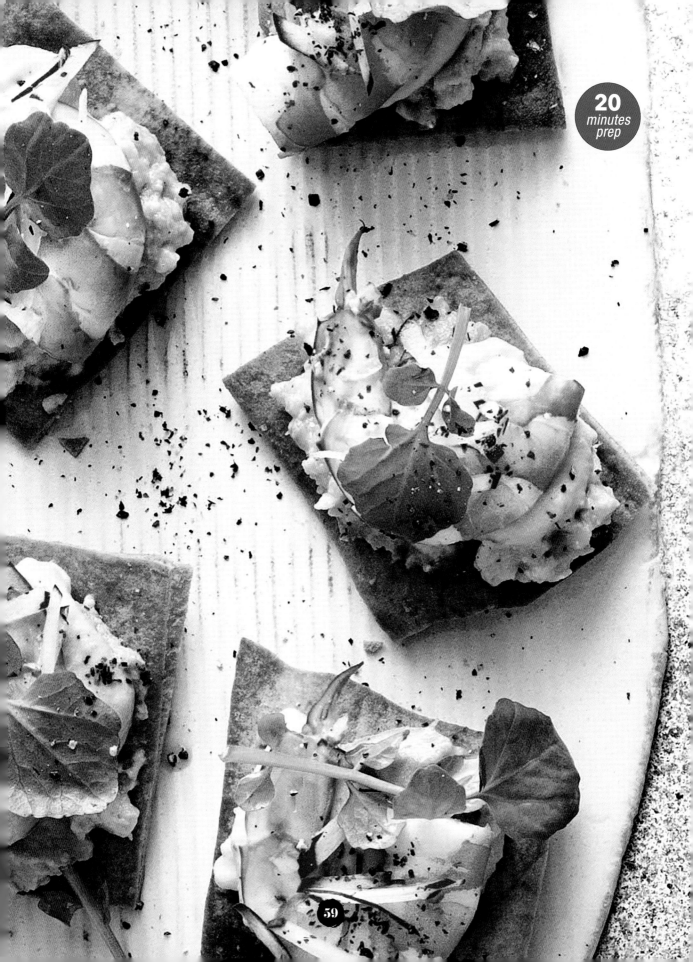

20
minutes
prep

59

Grilled Mushroom
BEEF KEBABS

This vegie-packed barbecue platter with beetroot and buckwheat salad makes a grillin' great light lunch with friends.

SERVES 6 **PREP** 30 mins (+ 1 hour marinating & 5 mins resting) **COOK** 25 mins

1 tbs finely chopped fresh
   rosemary leaves
60ml (¼ cup) extra virgin olive oil
80ml (⅓ cup) balsamic vinegar
3 garlic cloves, crushed
450g beef rump steak, excess fat
   trimmed, cut into 2cm pieces
250g cup mushrooms, halved
1 bunch baby beetroot, trimmed
205g (1 cup) buckwheat,
   rinsed, drained
250ml (1 cup) salt-reduced
   chicken stock
125ml (½ cup) fresh orange juice
1 cup fresh continental
   parsley leaves
½ small red onion, thinly sliced
2 tbs roughly chopped
   roasted hazelnuts
50g reduced-fat Greek feta,
   crumbled

1 Preheat oven to 200°C/180°C fan forced.

2 Combine the rosemary, 2 tbs oil, 2 tbs vinegar and two-thirds of the garlic in a large glass or ceramic bowl. Add the beef and mushroom. Stir until coated. Place in the fridge for 1 hour to marinate.

3 Meanwhile, wash the beetroot. Pat dry. Wrap individually in foil. Place on a baking tray. Roast for 40 minutes or until tender. Set aside until cool enough to handle. Wearing disposable gloves, peel the beetroot. Cut into wedges. Place the beetroot in a bowl. Add the remaining garlic and 1 tbs of the remaining vinegar. Season and toss to coat.

4 Heat a large saucepan over medium-high heat. Add the buckwheat. Cook, stirring, for 1 minute. Pour in the stock and orange juice. Stir to combine. Bring to the boil then reduce heat to medium. Simmer, covered, for 15-20 minutes or until the buckwheat is tender and liquid is absorbed. Remove from heat. Set aside for 5 minutes. Fluff the buckwheat with a fork. Transfer to a large bowl.

5 Preheat a barbecue grill or chargrill pan on medium-high. Thread the beef and mushroom onto metal or presoaked bamboo skewers. Cook for 2 minutes each side for medium or until cooked to your liking.

6 Add the parsley, onion, hazelnuts and feta to the buckwheat. Season and toss. Arrange the salad, beetroot and skewers on a serving platter. Whisk the remaining oil and vinegar in a small bowl. Drizzle over the salad and serve.

NUTRITION (PER SERVE)

CALS	FAT	SAT FAT	PROTEIN	CARBS
388	24.6g	4.1g	23.3g	28.9g

○ EASY   ○ QUICK   ● MAKE AHEAD   ○ MEAT FREE   ● FAMILY FRIENDLY

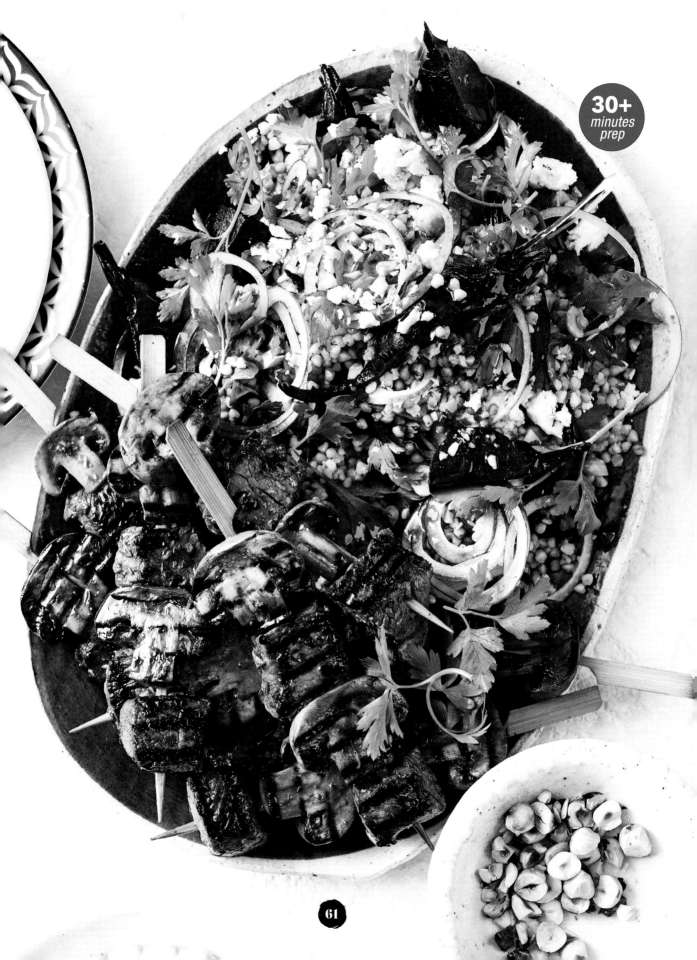

Tomato, Ricotta & Olive
SPELT TART

Healthier than shortcrust, the spelt pastry in this free-form tart is deliciously crisp. Swapping butter for olive oil adds a dose of heart-friendly fatty acids.

SERVES 6 **PREP** 25 mins (+ 30 mins resting) **COOK** 35 mins

½ cup fresh basil leaves, plus extra baby leaves to serve
½ cup fresh continental parsley leaves
2 tsp finely grated lemon rind
1 garlic clove, coarsely chopped
60g (⅓ cup) pitted Sicilian olives
2 tsp extra virgin olive oil
1 tsp fresh lemon juice
125g (½ cup) fresh ricotta
350g tomato medley mix, halved if large
150g mixed salad leaves (optional)
1 fennel bulb, thinly sliced (optional)
2 tsp balsamic vinegar (optional)

PASTRY
210g (1⅓ cups) white spelt flour
60ml (¼ cup) extra virgin olive oil
2 tbs finely grated parmesan
60ml (¼ cup) chilled water

1 To make the pastry, place the flour, oil and parmesan in a food processor and process until the mixture resembles fine crumbs. With the motor running, gradually add the chilled water until mixture just comes together. (Add 1-2 tsp extra, if necessary.) Shape into a disc. Wrap and place in the fridge for 30 minutes to rest. Clean the processor.
2 Preheat oven to 180°C/160°C fan forced.
3 Place the basil, parsley, lemon rind and garlic in the processor and process until finely chopped. Add the olives, oil and lemon juice. Process until well combined. Season.
4 Roll out the pastry on a large piece of baking paper to a 30-35cm circle. Transfer paper and pastry to a large baking tray. Spread half the olive mixture over the pastry base, leaving a 2cm border. Dollop with the ricotta and top with the tomato. Fold the pastry edge over the filling. Bake for 35 minutes or until the pastry is crisp.
5 Combine the salad leaves, fennel and vinegar in a bowl, if using. Top the tart with the remaining olive mixture and extra basil. Serve with the salad on the side.

COOK'S NOTE

Make the pastry up to 1 day in advance and store in plastic wrap in the fridge. The olive mixture can also be made a day ahead, making it quick and easy to assemble the tart and bake.

NUTRITION (PER SERVE)

CALS	FAT	SAT FAT	PROTEIN	CARBS
303	16g	4g	8g	29g

★★★★★

Love this recipe and it's pretty easy to make. **SABBIE13**

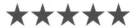

● EASY   ○ QUICK   ● MAKE AHEAD   ● MEAT FREE   ● FAMILY FRIENDLY

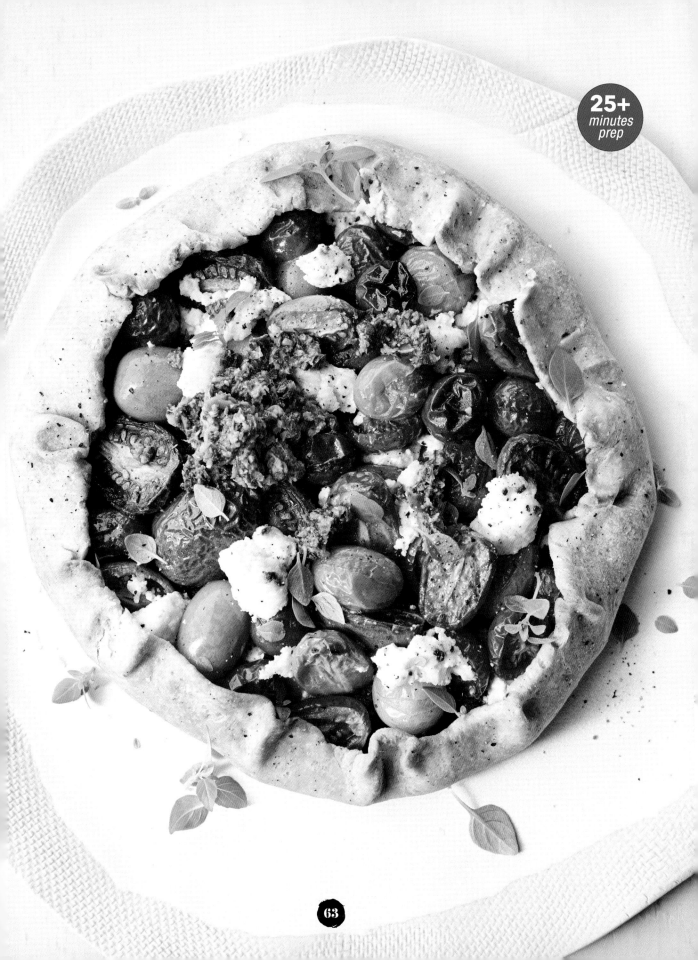

Quick Caper & Lemon TUNA BOWL

This no-cook lunch is a bit of everything we love about the Mediterranean diet all in one bowl – legumes, wholegrains, tuna and plenty of veg.

SERVES 4 **PREP** 20 mins

190g (1 cup) wholemeal couscous

250ml (1 cup) salt-reduced chicken stock, boiling

2 x 125g cans chickpeas, rinsed, drained

200g green beans

2 French shallots, finely chopped

1 tbs finely chopped capers

1 tsp finely grated lemon rind, plus extra rind, cut into thin strips, to serve

2 tbs fresh lemon juice

2 tbs extra virgin olive oil

425g can tuna in oil, drained, flaked

1 cup fresh continental parsley leaves

8 large iceberg lettuce leaves, torn

250g grape tomatoes, halved

180g tub mixed marinated olives

1 Place the couscous in a heatproof bowl. Add the stock. Stir. Cover and set aside for 5 minutes or until all the liquid is absorbed. Use a fork to separate the grains then stir in the chickpeas.

2 Meanwhile, place the beans in a heatproof bowl. Cover with boiling water. Set aside for 2 minutes to blanch. Drain and refresh under cold running water.

3 Combine the shallot, capers, lemon rind and juice, and oil in a small bowl. Season. Place the tuna in a separate bowl. Add half the dressing and half the parsley. Toss to combine.

4 Spoon the couscous mixture into serving bowls. Top with the lettuce, beans, tomato, olives and tuna mixture. Sprinkle with the remaining parsley and extra lemon rind. Drizzle over the remaining dressing to serve.

COOK'S NOTE

Make extra of this zesty dish and take the leftovers to work the next day.

NUTRITION (PER SERVE)

CALS	FAT	SAT FAT	PROTEIN	CARBS
582	25.5g	3.9g	33.2g	61.4g

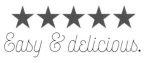

★★★★★

Easy & delicious.

STEWARTK999

● EASY ● QUICK ● MAKE AHEAD ○ MEAT FREE ○ FAMILY FRIENDLY

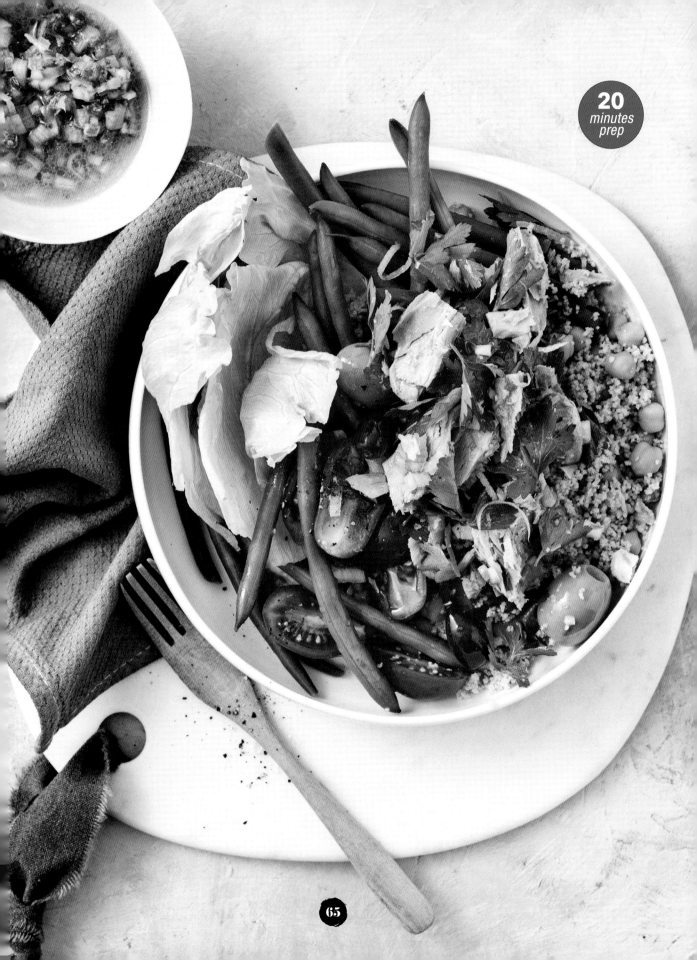

20
minutes
prep

65

Mushroom & Feta CAPSICUM WRAPS

Load up wraps with roasted and sauteed vegetables for a quick and easy power lunch. Enjoy a vitamin C and betacarotene hit thanks to the capsicums.

SERVES 4 **PREP** 10 mins **COOK** 15 mins

8 portobello mushrooms
3 tsp extra virgin olive oil
2 garlic cloves, crushed
1 red onion, thinly sliced
1 red capsicum, deseeded,
    thinly sliced
1 yellow capsicum, deseeded,
    thinly sliced
2 tbs chopped fresh continental
    parsley leaves
4 wholegrain wraps, warmed
80g baby spinach
½ avocado, mashed
50g Greek feta, crumbled

1 Preheat the grill on high. Line a baking tray with foil.
2 Place the mushrooms, cup-side up, on prepared tray. Combine 2 tsp oil and half the garlic in a small bowl. Brush the garlic mixture over the mushroom cups to coat. Grill, turning halfway through, for 6-8 minutes or until the mushrooms are golden and tender.
3 Meanwhile, heat the remaining 1 tsp oil in a large non-stick frying pan over medium-high heat. Add the onion and cook, stirring, for 5 minutes or until tender. Add the capsicum and remaining garlic. Cook, stirring, for 10 minutes or until the mixture starts to caramelise. Stir in the parsley.
4 Cut the grilled mushrooms in half. Top each wrap with the spinach, capsicum mixture and mushroom. Add a dollop of the mashed avocado. Sprinkle with the feta. Fold up to enclose and serve.

COOK'S NOTE

For a twist, turn this into a salad. Omit the wraps, increase the spinach to a 120g bag and serve in a large salad bowl.

NUTRITION (PER SERVE)

CALS	FAT	SAT FAT	PROTEIN	CARBS
322	16g	5g	13g	26g

★★★★★

I thought these were delicious, especially with the feta giving it a nice tang.
GABRIELE650GS

● EASY ● QUICK ○ MAKE AHEAD ● MEAT FREE ● FAMILY FRIENDLY

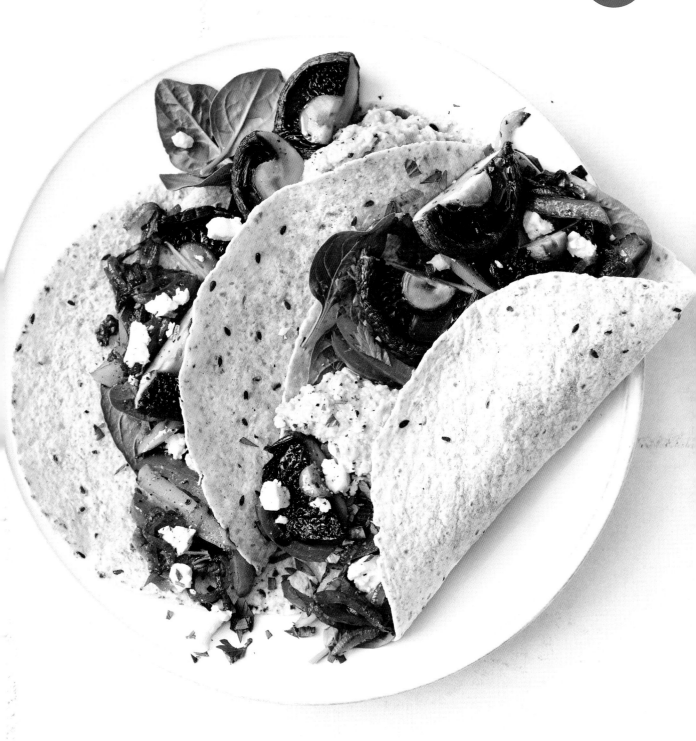

Easy Couscous
SEAFOOD PARCELS

A novel little parcel to open, the whole family will 'oooh' and 'aaah' when they open up this healthy, super veg and seafood surprise.

SERVES 4 **PREP** 15 mins **COOK** 20 mins

240g skinless salmon fillet, cut into 2cm pieces

200g green prawns, peeled, deveined, tails intact

250g cherry tomatoes, halved

2 small zucchini, thinly sliced

50g (⅓ cup) pitted Sicilian olives, sliced

2 tsp finely grated lemon rind

80ml (⅓ cup) salt-reduced vegetable stock

90g (½ cup) wholemeal couscous

125ml (½ cup) boiling water

150g sugar snap peas

150g snow peas

1 Preheat oven to 200°C/180°C fan forced. Tear four 30cm squares of foil and four 30cm squares of baking paper.
2 Combine the salmon, prawns, tomato, zucchini, olives and lemon rind in a large bowl. Place 1 piece of baking paper on top of 1 piece of foil. Place one-quarter of the salmon mixture in the centre of the baking paper. Pour over 1 tbs stock. Fold up the foil to enclose the filling. Place on a large baking tray. Repeat with the remaining baking paper and foil squares, salmon mixture and stock to create 4 parcels in total. Bake for 12-15 minutes or until the salmon flakes easily when tested with a fork.
3 Meanwhile, place the couscous in a heatproof bowl. Pour over the boiling water. Stir to combine. Cover and set aside for 3 minutes or until the liquid is absorbed. Use a fork to separate the grains. Season.
4 Cook the sugar snap peas and snow peas in a saucepan of boiling water for 2-3 minutes or until bright green and tender crisp. Drain.
5 Serve the parcels with the sugar snap peas, snow peas and couscous.

COOK'S NOTE

Not a fan of prawns? Leave them out and double the salmon. The peas could be swapped with green beans or broccoli florets.

NUTRITION (PER SERVE)

CALS	FAT	SAT FAT	PROTEIN	CARBS
325	12g	2.2g	30.2g	19.9g

● EASY ○ QUICK ○ MAKE AHEAD ○ MEAT FREE ● FAMILY FRIENDLY

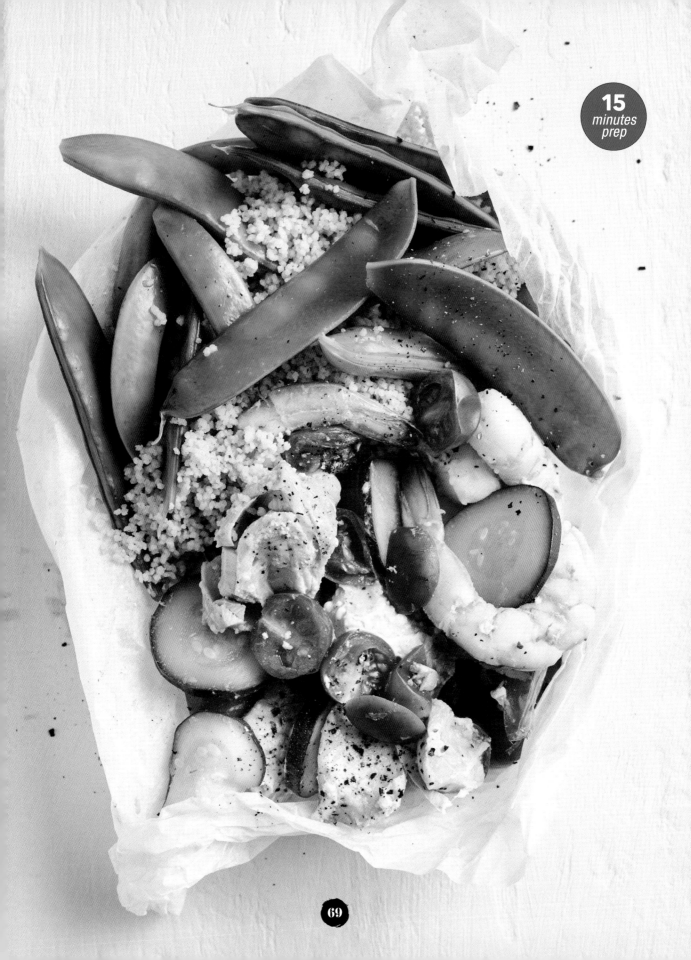

15
minutes
prep

Tahini & Kale
RED LENTIL PENNE

Welcome legumes to the pasta party for a wholesome boost! Toss through a heavenly tahini and garlic dressing for the ultimate flavour bomb.

SERVES 6 **PREP** 20 mins **COOK** 45 mins

½ (about 900g) butternut pumpkin, peeled, deseeded, cut into 1.5cm pieces
1 tbs extra virgin olive oil
½ tsp cumin seeds, crushed
¼ tsp dried chilli flakes
2 cups kale leaves
250g red lentil pasta
Black sesame seeds, to sprinkle (optional)

TAHINI DRESSING
80ml (⅓ cup) tahini
2 tbs extra virgin olive oil
2 tbs fresh lemon juice
3 tsp apple cider vinegar
1 garlic clove, crushed
60ml (¼ cup) warm water
¼ cup finely chopped fresh coriander leaves

1 Preheat oven to 200°C/180°C fan forced. Grease 2 baking trays and line with baking paper.
2 Place the pumpkin on 1 tray. Season with salt. Drizzle over the oil. Roast, turning occasionally, for 25 minutes or until it starts to turn golden. Sprinkle with cumin and chilli.
3 Place the kale on remaining prepared tray and spray with extra virgin olive oil. Return the pumpkin to oven along with the kale. Roast for 10 minutes or until the pumpkin is golden and kale is crispy.
4 Meanwhile, make the dressing. Combine the tahini, oil, lemon juice, vinegar and garlic in a small jug (don't worry if the mixture seizes). Stir in the warm water until the mixture loosens again. Add the coriander, season and stir to combine.
5 Cook the pasta in a large saucepan of boiling water following packet directions or until al dente. Add 1 tbs of the cooking liquid to the dressing. Stir to combine. Drain the pasta. Transfer to a large bowl. Toss through three-quarters of the dressing. Serve the pasta topped with pumpkin, kale, remaining dressing and sesame seeds, if using.

COOK'S NOTE

Roast the pumpkin up to 1 day ahead. Cover and refrigerate, then warm in the microwave before using. The dressing can be made up to a day head. Keep in a jar in the fridge. Return to room temperature

NUTRITION (PER SERVE)

CALS	FAT	SAT FAT	PROTEIN	CARBS
373	23.5g	2.5g	11g	35g

● EASY ○ QUICK ● MAKE AHEAD ● MEAT FREE ○ FAMILY FRIENDLY

★★★★★

I wasn't initially convinced when I tried the sauce, but it worked well with the red lentil pasta and the vegetables, especially the chilli. **PCLARK**

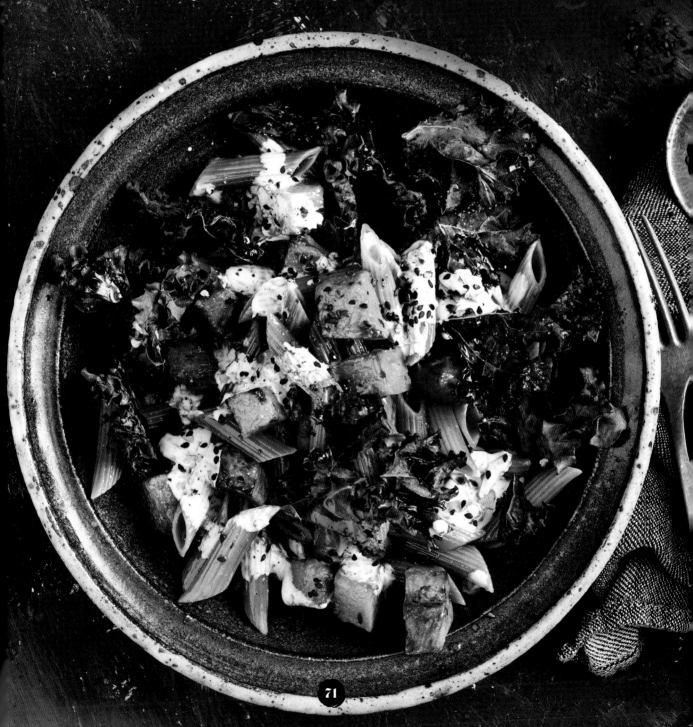

20 minutes prep

Prawn & Avocado RADICCHIO CUPS

Attack snacktime with radicchio and watercress – they're nutrient powerhouses that pair so well with prawns and a herby avo vinaigrette.

SERVES 4 **PREP** 20 mins

1 small radicchio lettuce,
  leaves separated
1 small bunch watercress,
  sprigs picked
24 cooked king prawns, peeled,
  deveined, tails intact
Lemon cheeks, to serve
AVOCADO VINAIGRETTE
1 ripe avocado
2 green shallots, finely chopped
½ cup fresh coriander leaves
¼ cup fresh mint leaves
¼ cup fresh dill
1 garlic clove
1 lemon, rind finely grated (see note)
2 tbs extra virgin olive oil
1 tsp apple cider vinegar
1-2 tbs fresh lemon juice,
  to taste

1 To make the avocado vinaigrette, place the avocado, shallot, coriander, mint, dill, garlic and lemon rind in a food processor or high-powered blender. Process until finely chopped. Add the oil, vinegar and lemon juice. Process until smooth and creamy. Season. Add 3-4 tbs water, if you prefer a runnier consistency, then blend until smooth
2 Arrange the radicchio leaves on serving plates. Top with the watercress and prawns. Drizzle over the avocado vinaigrette and serve with lemon cheeks to squeeze over.

NUTRITION (PER SERVE)

CALS	FAT	SAT FAT	PROTEIN	CARBS
285	19g	4g	26g	2g

COOK'S NOTE

Juice the lemon that you've grated the rind from for the avocado vinaigrette. Drizzle the vinaigrette over your favourite salad or use as a dip for vegie sticks. Store in the fridge and use within 2 days.

★★★★★

Surprised how creamy the dressing was thanks just to the avocado. I ate this totally guilt free! **FANCY FOODIE**

● EASY   ● QUICK   ○ MAKE AHEAD   ○ MEAT FREE   ● FAMILY FRIENDLY

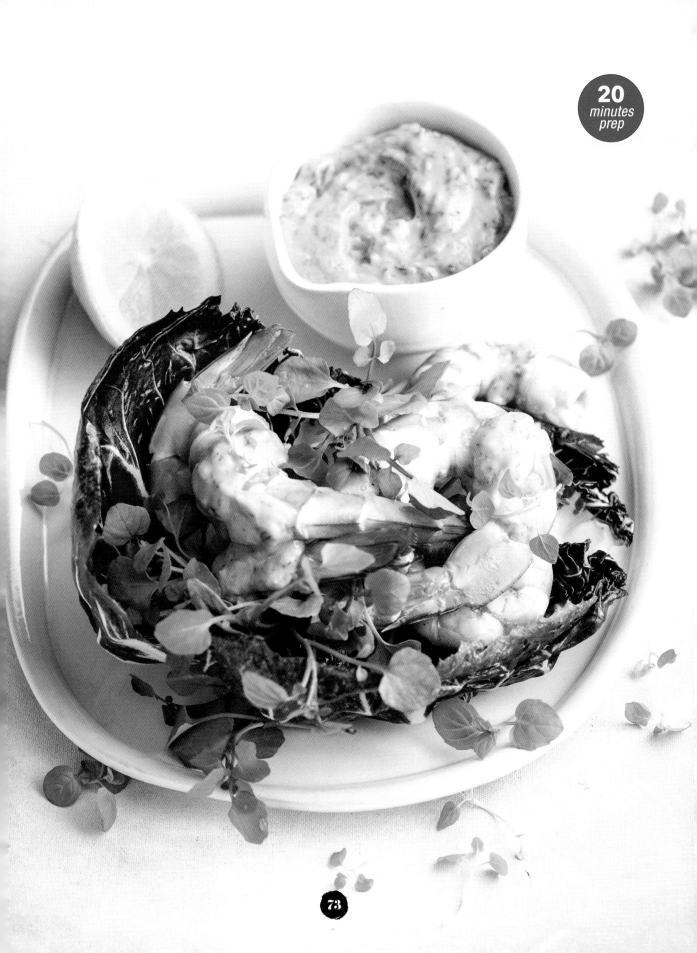

20
minutes
prep

73

Crudité & Herbed
YOGHURT DIP

Dip and crunch your way through this nibbly. Just serve this super easy, four ingredient-dip with your favourite vegie sticks or other dippers.

SERVES 6 **PREP** 10 mins

1 garlic clove, crushed

1 tsp finely grated lemon rind, plus extra to serve

⅓ cup chopped mixed fresh herb leaves (such as mint, parsley and chives), plus extra to serve

390g (1½ cups) reduced-fat Greek-style yoghurt

Raw vegetables (such as baby corn, baby carrots and radishes), to serve

1 Place the garlic, lemon rind, herbs and yoghurt in a bowl. Season and stir to combine.

2 Transfer the dip to a serving bowl. Sprinkle with extra herbs and lemon rind. Serve with vegetables.

NUTRITION (PER SERVE)

CALS	FAT	SAT FAT	PROTEIN	CARBS
89	2.4g	1.4g	3.9g	11.7g

COOK'S NOTE

Store any leftover dip in an airtight container in the fridge for up to 5 days. This is also delicious as a spread for sandwiches and wraps instead of butter.

★★★★★

This recipe was simple to make and was very tasty and refreshing.

CAZ65

● EASY ● QUICK ● MAKE AHEAD ● MEAT FREE ● FAMILY FRIENDLY

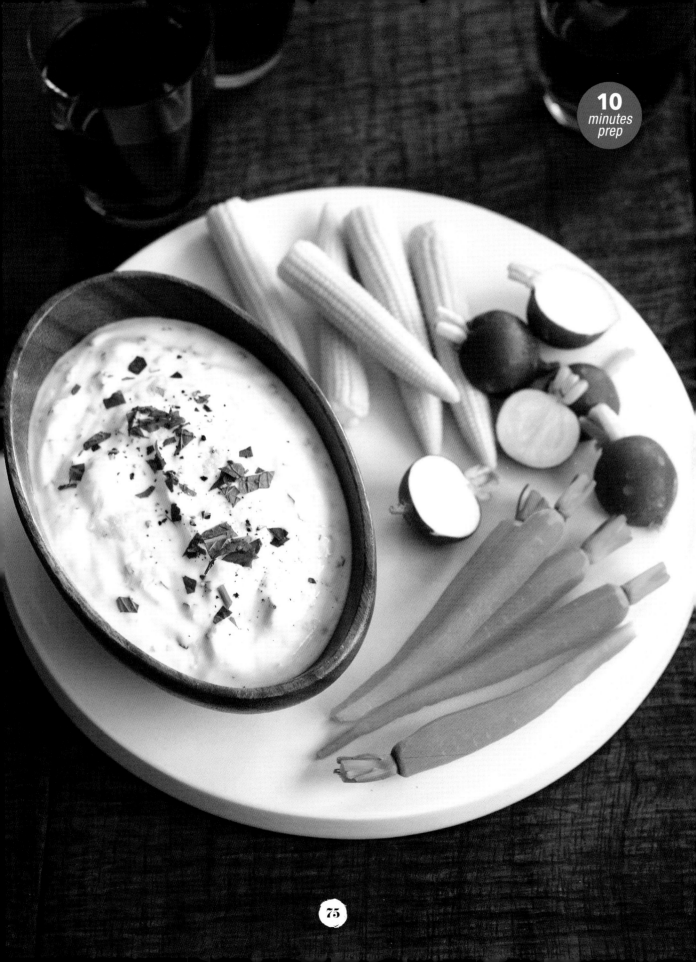

Green Tahini
LAMB MEATBALLS

We've jammed even more veg into this colourful dish by adding spinach to the zesty tahini dressing. Time to start rollin' those meatballs!

SERVES 6 **PREP** 10 mins **COOK** 25 mins

8 baby carrots, unpeeled, trimmed, scrubbed, halved lengthways

2 large beetroots, trimmed, scrubbed, cut into thin wedges

2 small red onions, cut into thin wedges

1 red capsicum, deseeded, thickly sliced

80ml (⅓ cup) extra virgin olive oil, plus extra to drizzle

425g can no-added-salt lentils, rinsed, drained

500g lamb mince

2 tsp ground cumin

2 tsp ground coriander

60ml (¼ cup) fresh lemon juice

2 tbs tahini

120g baby spinach

1 Preheat oven to 220°C/200°C fan forced. Line a baking tray with baking paper.

2 Place the carrot, beetroot, onion and capsicum on prepared tray. Drizzle over 2 tbs oil and toss until coated. Roast for 25 minutes or until tender. Add the lentils and toss until heated through.

3 Meanwhile, place the lamb, cumin and coriander in a large bowl. Season and mix until well combined. Roll level tablespoonfuls of the mixture into balls. Heat 1 tbs of the remaining oil in a large frying pan over medium-high heat. Cook the meatballs, turning, for 8 minutes or until browned and cooked through. Transfer to plate.

4 Place the lemon juice, tahini, 2 tbs water, remaining oil and half the spinach in a small food processor. Process until smooth. Season. Divide among serving plates. Top with the roast vegetable mixture, meatballs and remaining spinach. Drizzle over extra oil. Season with pepper to serve.

COOK'S NOTE

Make this super speedy by using pre-chopped roasting veg – find them in the fruit and veg section at the supermarket. Serve with wholemeal flatbread, if you like.

NUTRITION (PER SERVE)

CALS	FAT	SAT FAT	PROTEIN	CARBS
387	24g	4.7g	24g	15.1g

★★★★★

Easy and tasty, highly recommend giving this one a go! **JAPAJO**

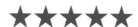 ● EASY ○ QUICK ○ MAKE AHEAD ○ MEAT FREE ● FAMILY FRIENDLY

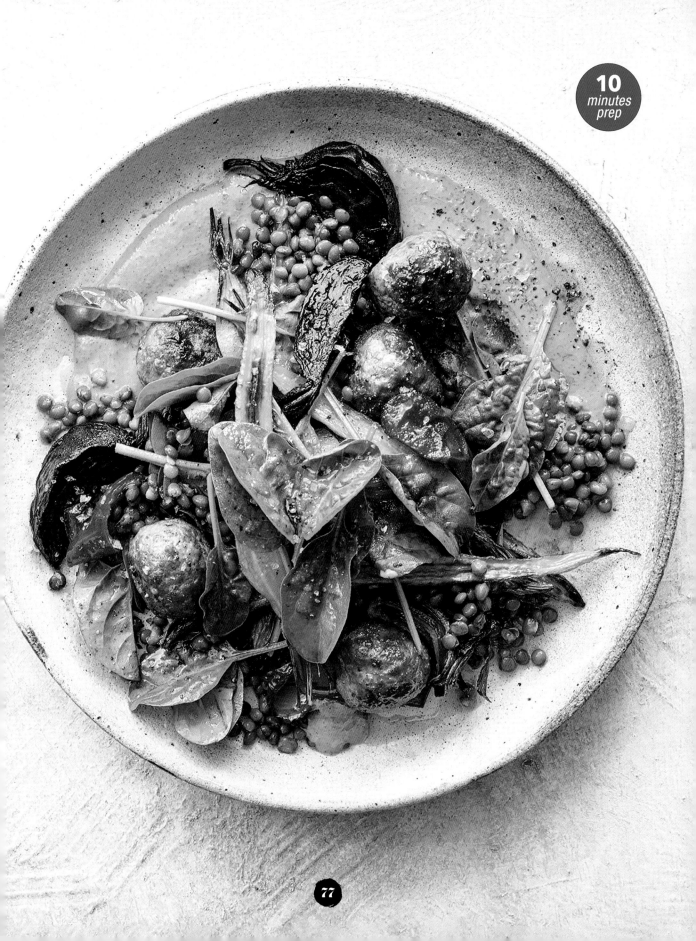

Chilli Tuna & Rocket
BRUSCHETTA

Load up freshly sliced sourdough with spiced tuna, tomatoes and rocket for a quick 15-minute meal or prep ahead and eat al desko.

SERVES 4 **PREP** 15 mins

425g can tuna in spring water, drained, flaked
250g cherry tomatoes, halved
½ cup chopped fresh continental parsley leaves
2 tbs fresh lemon juice
1 tbs extra virgin olive oil
Large pinch of dried chilli flakes
8 slices wholemeal sourdough bread
80g baby rocket

1 Combine the tuna, tomato, parsley, lemon juice, oil and chilli in a bowl.
2 Place the bread on serving plates. Top with the rocket and tuna mixture.

NUTRITION (PER SERVE)

CALS	FAT	SAT FAT	PROTEIN	CARBS
295	8g	2g	28g	24g

COOK'S NOTE

Prepare the tuna mixture the night before and store in individual airtight containers in the fridge. Assemble at work.

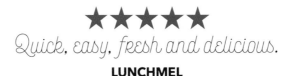

★★★★★
Quick, easy, fresh and delicious.
LUNCHMEL

● EASY ● QUICK ● MAKE AHEAD ○ MEAT FREE ○ FAMILY FRIENDLY

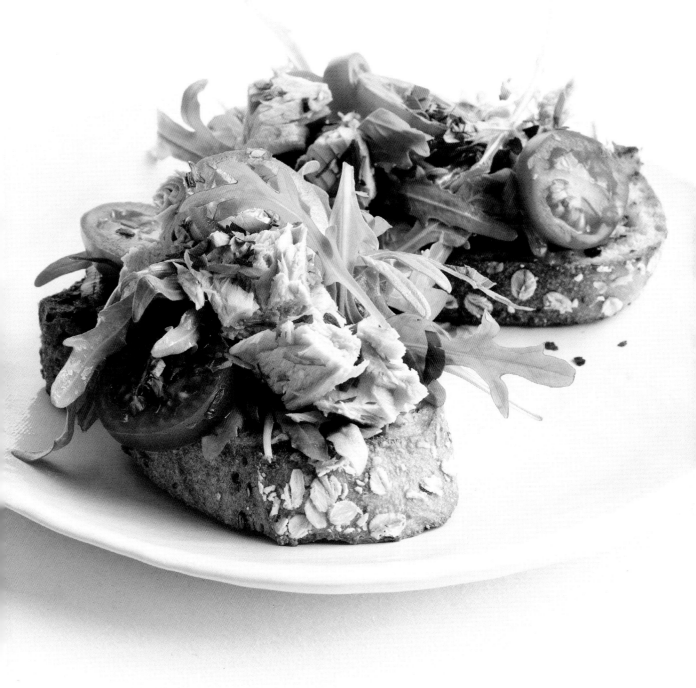

15
minutes
prep

Greek Baked
EGGPLANT

Get a taste of the Med with this classic Greek dish. The eggplant is salted and grilled, then slowly baked in a fresh tomato sauce.

SERVES 6 **PREP** 35 mins (+ 30 mins resting) **COOK** 1 hour

3 medium eggplants
125ml (½ cup) extra virgin olive oil
1 brown onion, finely chopped
2 garlic cloves, crushed
6 vine ripened tomatoes, peeled, deseeded, chopped (see note)
2 tbs tomato paste
1 tbs chopped fresh basil leaves, plus extra baby leaves to serve
2 tsp brown sugar
150g Greek feta, crumbled
Micro herbs, to serve

1 Cut the eggplants in half lengthways. Score the flesh in a crosshatch pattern. Season with salt. Set aside for 30 minutes to soften slightly.
2 Meanwhile, heat 2 tbs oil in a large saucepan over medium heat. Add the onion. Cook, stirring, for 10 minutes or until softened. Add the garlic. Stir for 1 minute or until aromatic. Add the tomato, tomato paste, basil, sugar and 125ml (½ cup) water. Bring to the boil. Reduce heat to low and simmer, stirring occasionally, for 20 minutes or until thickened. Season.
3 Preheat oven to 200°C/180°C fan forced. Spray a large baking dish with extra virgin olive oil.
4 Rinse the eggplant under cold running water. Pat dry. Heat half the remaining oil in a large frying pan over medium heat. Add half the eggplant and cook, cut-side down, for 5-8 minutes or until golden. Transfer to prepared dish. Repeat with the remaining oil and eggplant.
5 Spoon the tomato mixture over the eggplant. Cover the dish with foil. Roast for 30 minutes or until the eggplant is tender. Top with the feta. Roast, uncovered, for 10 minutes or until golden. Top with extra basil and micro herbs to serve.

COOK'S NOTE

To peel tomatoes, cut a shallow cross in base of each one. Place in a saucepan of boiling water for 5 seconds. Transfer to a bowl of cold water. Set aside for 1 minute then peel skin. Halve horizontally and scoop out seeds with a teaspoon. Serve this dish with wholemeal sourdough or pita bread, if you like.

NUTRITION (PER SERVE)

CALS	FAT	SAT FAT	PROTEIN	CARBS
333	25.5g	6.5g	8.2g	13.9g

● EASY ○ QUICK ○ MAKE AHEAD ● MEAT FREE ● FAMILY FRIENDLY

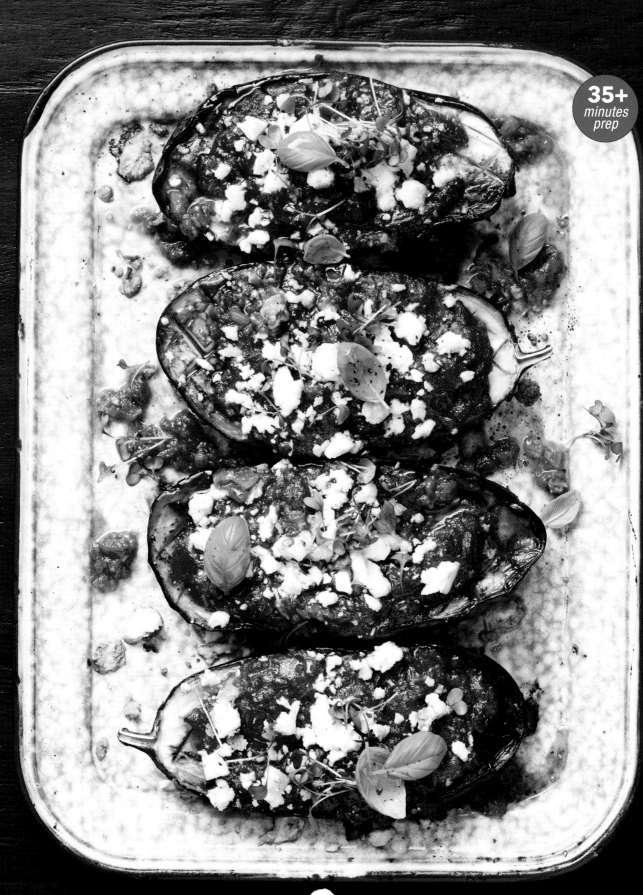

Dukkah-Swirled
LABNE DIP

Have you made labne before? It's as easy as leaving yoghurt overnight to drain in the fridge. It makes a delicious dip – just add salt, dukkah and olive oil.

SERVES 8 **PREP** 10 mins (+ overnight draining)

500g Greek-style yoghurt
1 tsp sea salt flakes
2 tbs almond, lemon and
   herb dukkah
1 tbs extra virgin olive oil
Thin strips of lemon rind, to serve
Wholegrain crispbreads and
   vegetables (such as radishes and
   green beans), to serve (optional)

1 Combine the yoghurt and salt in a bowl. Line a sieve with 2 layers of muslin cloth. (Alternatively, use 5 layers of paper towel.) Set prepared sieve over a bowl. Spoon the yoghurt mixture into the sieve. Cover and place in the fridge overnight to drain the excess liquid from the yoghurt.
2 Transfer the labne to a serving bowl, discarding the drained liquid. Swirl through the dukkah. Drizzle over the oil and sprinkle with lemon rind. Season and serve with crispbreads and vegetables, if using.

COOK'S NOTE

The labne will keep, covered, in the fridge for up to 1 week. It is also fab on fresh wholegrain sourdough drizzled with honey or dolloped on a baked potato instead of sour cream.

NUTRITION (PER SERVE)

CALS	FAT	SAT FAT	PROTEIN	CARBS
129	10.3g	4.2g	4.4g	4.4g

★★★★★

I made this for an antipasto and dip platter for a party. It worked so well, and making it the day before really helped on the day.

WAFFLEISO

● EASY   ○ QUICK   ● MAKE AHEAD   ● MEAT FREE   ● FAMILY FRIENDLY

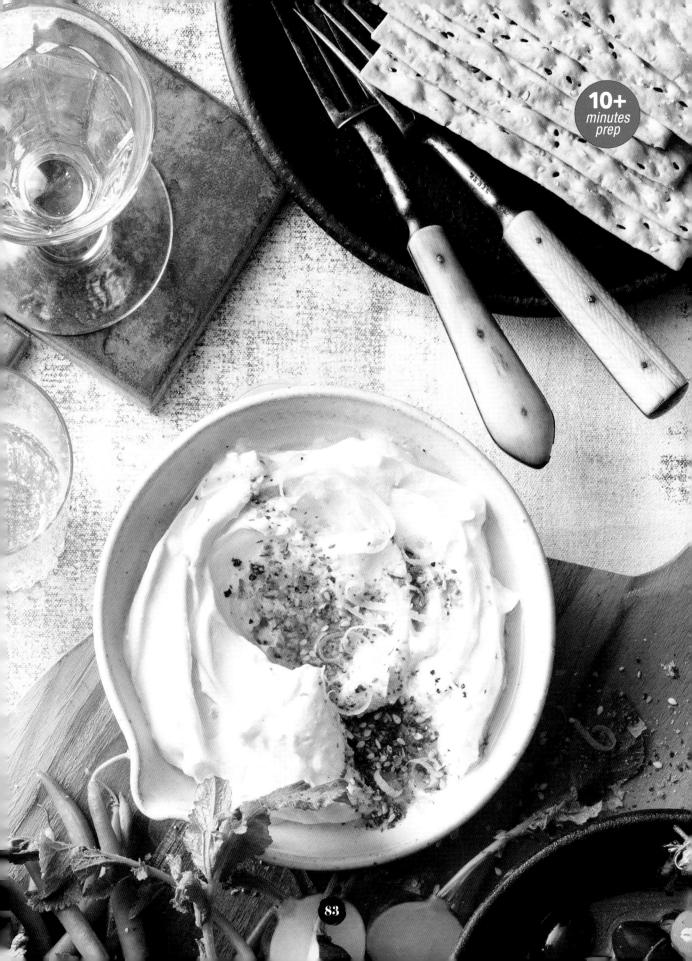

10+
minutes
prep

Healthy Chilli
TUNA PATTIES

Canned tuna is an easy, budget way to eat more seafood. Use it and loads of vegies to pack your patties with immunity-boosting goodness.

SERVES 4 **PREP** 20 mins (+ cooling) **COOK** 20 mins

1 large red capsicum,
  halved, deseeded
1½ tbs extra virgin olive oil
1 large carrot, peeled,
  coarsely grated
150g green beans, thinly sliced
1 tsp ground cumin
2 eggs
40g (¼ cup) wholemeal spelt flour
185g can tuna in chilli olive oil,
  drained, flaked
175g (1 cup) cooked quinoa
  (see note)
⅓ cup chopped fresh continental
  parsley leaves, plus 2 tbs extra
90g (⅓ cup) Greek-style yoghurt
1 tbs fresh lemon juice
350g pkt cranberry and
  kale slaw kit
Lemon wedges, to serve

1 Finely chop 1 capsicum half. Thinly slice the remaining half. Heat 1 tsp oil in a large non-stick frying pan over medium heat. Add the chopped capsicum, carrot and beans. Cook, stirring, for 1 minute. Add the cumin. Cook, stirring, for 2 minutes or until the vegetables are just tender. Set aside to cool.
2 Whisk together the eggs and flour in a large bowl until well combined. Add the tuna, quinoa, parsley and cooled vegetables. Season and stir until combined. Shape the mixture into 12 patties. Clean the pan.
3 Heat the remaining oil in the pan over medium-high heat. Cook the patties, in batches if necessary, for 2-3 minutes each side or until golden.
4 Meanwhile, combine the yoghurt, lemon juice and extra parsley in a small bowl. Combine the slaw kit (reserve the dressing for another use), reserved sliced capsicum and a little yoghurt dressing in a large bowl.
5 Serve the patties with the slaw, yoghurt dressing and lemon wedges to squeeze over.

COOK'S NOTE

To make 175g (1 cup) cooked quinoa, use about 55g (¼ cup) uncooked.

NUTRITION (PER SERVE)

CALS	FAT	SAT FAT	PROTEIN	CARBS
306	14.1g	3g	18g	22.2g

★★★★★

Quick, healthy and easy for a midweek dinner. **ALISHA**

● **EASY** ○ QUICK ○ MAKE AHEAD ○ MEAT FREE ○ FAMILY FRIENDLY

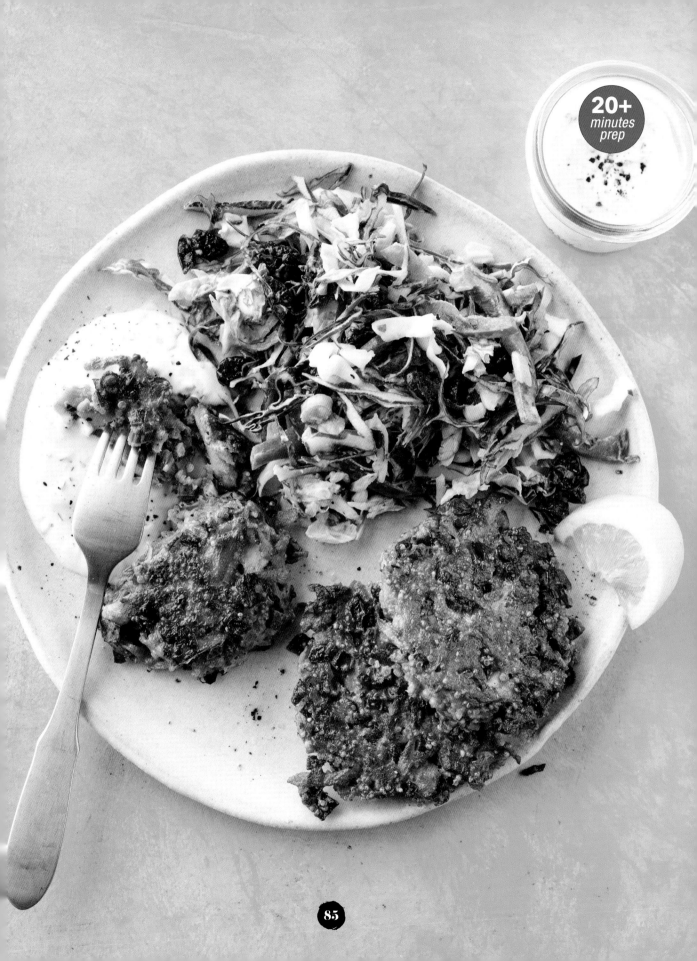

20+
minutes
prep

Classic Herby
ARTICHOKES

One artichoke is enough to give you 20 per cent of your daily vitamin C!
Celebrate with this Roman-style braised dish, known as carciofi alla romana.

MAKES 4 **PREP** 40 mins **COOK** 40 mins

1 lemon, halved
4 globe artichokes
⅓ cup chopped fresh continental
    parsley leaves
2 tbs chopped fresh mint leaves
2 garlic cloves, finely chopped
2 tbs extra virgin olive oil, plus
    185ml (¾ cup) extra
125ml (½ cup) white wine
Micro herbs, to serve

1 Fill a bowl with water. Squeeze in the juice of 1 lemon half. Trim the large stalk of 1 artichoke until 5cm long. Starting at the base and spinning the artichoke around, snap off the thick green leaves, down to the white part, rubbing cuts with the remaining lemon half (continue rubbing cuts with lemon as you prepare the artichokes).
2 Use a sharp knife to cut about 3cm (about one-third, depending how big the artichoke is) from artichoke top to reveal a circle of purple-coloured leaves. Use a paring knife to cut around these leaves to reveal the choke (a cluster of silky thin purple and white 'hairs'). Use a spoon to scrape out the fuzzy choke. Use the knife to scrape back the stem and underside to reveal the white heart. Place in the bowl of lemon water. Repeat with the remaining artichokes.
3 Combine the parsley, mint and garlic in a bowl. Season. Stir in the oil.
4 Pat dry the artichokes then loosen the leaves. Stuff with the parsley mixture. Place the artichokes, stem-side up, in a saucepan. Pour in the wine and extra oil. Pour in enough water to reach one-third of the way up the sides of the artichoke leaves (not the stem). Cover with 2 layers of baking paper and the lid. Simmer for 40 minutes or until tender.
5 Use tongs to transfer the artichokes to a serving plate. Drizzle over some of the cooking liquid and sprinkle with micro herbs.

COOK'S NOTE

Go for artichokes that are tightly packed and have crisp green or purple leaves with a slight bloom. They should feel heavy for their size and 'squeak' when gently squeezed.

NUTRITION (EACH)

CALS	FAT	SAT FAT	PROTEIN	CARBS
220	18.7g	2.9g	4.1g	2.3g

○ EASY ○ QUICK ● MAKE AHEAD ● MEAT FREE ○ FAMILY FRIENDLY

40
minutes
prep

★★★★★

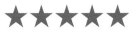
I can never go past anything artichoke!

DRPRETTY

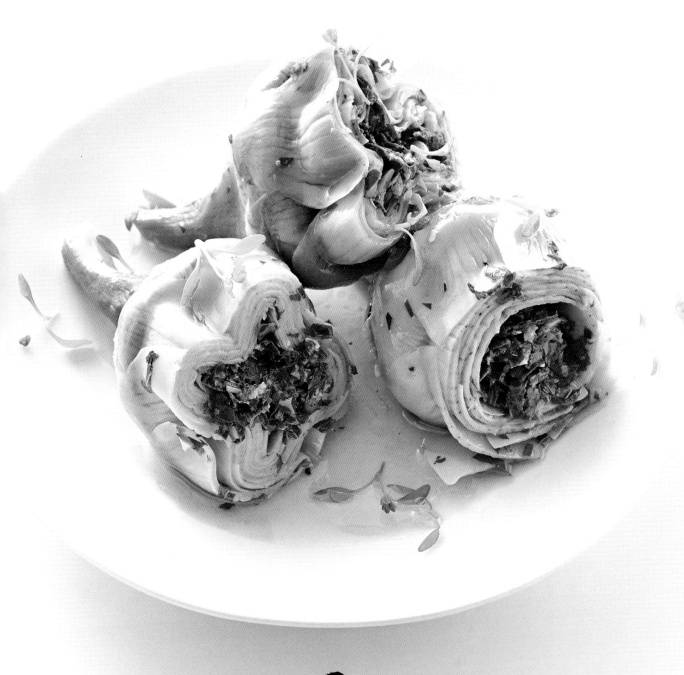

Slow Cooker Stuffed
CAPSICUMS

Put your slow cooker to work, no matter what time of year it is. Stuffed with currants and brown rice, these caps are amazing when cooked low and slow.

SERVES 6 **PREP** 20 mins **COOK** 4 hours

8 small red, yellow and
   green capsicums
250g pkt microwave brown rice
80ml (⅓ cup) passata
55g (⅓ cup) currants
2 green shallots, thinly sliced
2 tbs extra virgin olive oil
Greek-style yoghurt, fresh coriander
   leaves and pomegranate arils,
   to serve

1 Lightly grease the bowl of a slow cooker and line with baking paper. Cut the tops off the capsicums and discard. Remove the seeds and membrane.
2 Combine the rice, passata, currants, shallot and 60ml (¼ cup) water in a bowl. Season well. Divide the mixture among the capsicums. Place the capsicums, cut-side up, in prepared slow cooker. Drizzle over the oil, cover and cook on High for 4 hours or until the capsicums are soft.
3 Serve the stuffed capsicums topped with yoghurt, coriander and pomegranate.

COOK'S NOTE

Change up the filling, if you like. Try chopped zucchini and chilli for a spicy kick.

NUTRITION (PER SERVE)

CALS	FAT	SAT FAT	PROTEIN	CARBS
235	8.9g	1.8g	6.7g	29.1g

★★★★★

I've made these a few times. First as a side for the fam to try, but they were so popular it became a main! I kept the tops and served them like mini cloches – the kids loved that! **VIOLAPARMESAN**

● EASY   ○ QUICK   ○ MAKE AHEAD   ● MEAT FREE   ● FAMILY FRIENDLY

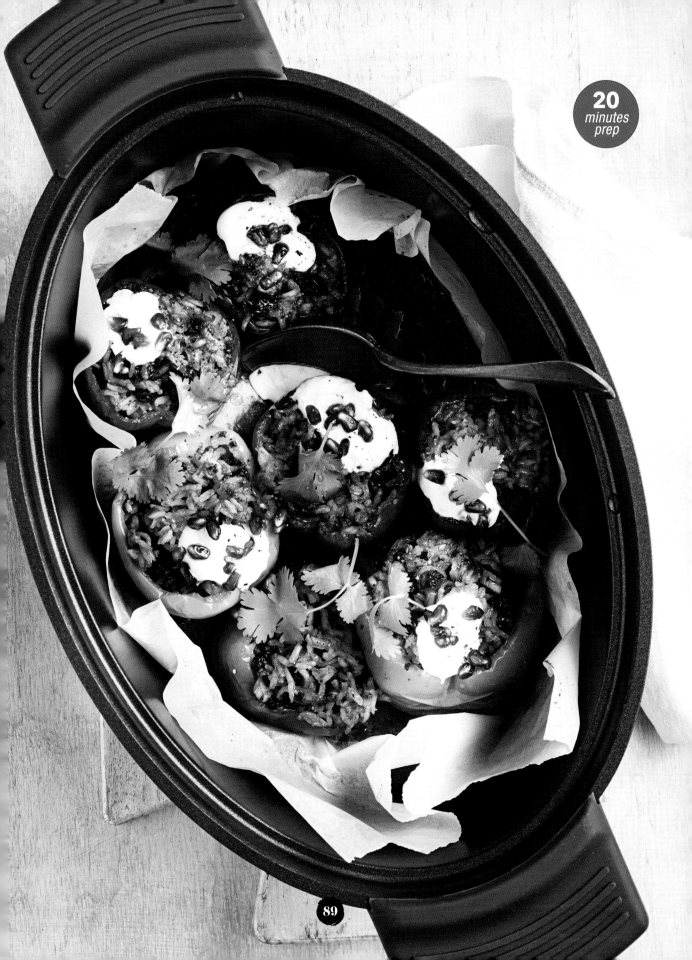

Kale Slaw SARDINE TOASTS

This bruschetta is ready in 10 minutes, perfect for lunch on the go or a light dinner when all you want to do is flop on the couch.

SERVES 4 **PREP** 5 mins **COOK** 5 mins

300g (4 cups) kale slaw kit
4 small tomatoes, deseeded, coarsely chopped
2 tbs fresh lemon juice
4 wholemeal sandwich thins, halved, toasted
4 x 105g cans sardines in olive oil, drained (see note)
Lemon wedges, to serve

1 Combine the kale slaw (reserve the dressing for another use), tomato and lemon juice in a small bowl. Season.
2 Top the sandwich thins with the kale mixture and sardines. Serve with lemon wedges to squeeze over.

NUTRITION (PER SERVE)

CALS	FAT	SAT FAT	PROTEIN	CARBS
338	14g	4g	24g	25g

COOK'S NOTE

Swap the sardines for canned tuna or salmon in olive oil, if you prefer.

★★★★★

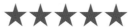

Pre-chopped bag of salad put to the very best use!

FRIDGETUNER

● EASY   ● QUICK   ○ MAKE AHEAD   ○ MEAT FREE   ○ FAMILY FRIENDLY

5
minutes
prep

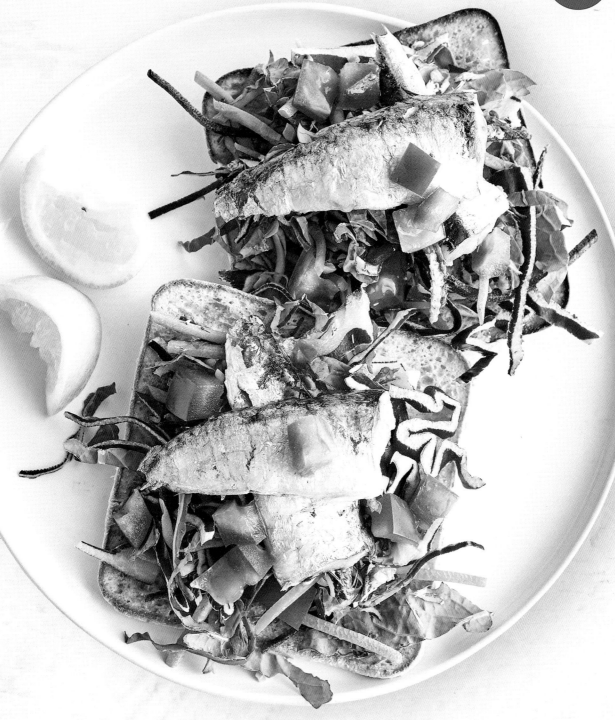

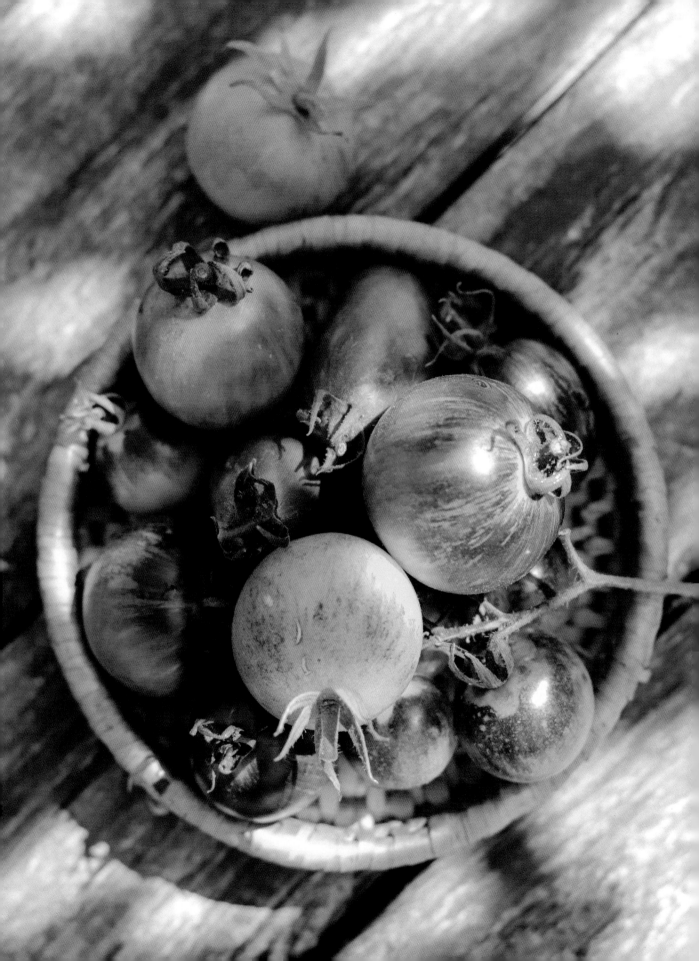

SALADS

THE MEDITERRANEAN DIET HAS A BIG FOCUS ON
PLANT-BASED EATING, SO TUCK INTO A BOUNTY
OF FRESH PRODUCE TO START ENJOYING
ALL THE AMAZING BENEFITS!

Dukkah
CHICKPEA CRUNCH

This is our idea of crunch time! Crispy, dukkah-spiced chickpeas tossed with green beans, radishes and gem lettuce, it's simple yet effective.

SERVES 4 (as a side) **PREP** 10 mins **COOK** 10 mins

2 x 125g cans chickpeas,
    drained, rinsed
2 tbs extra virgin olive oil
2 tbs lemon and herb dukkah
200g green beans
80g (½ cup) frozen peas
2 tbs fresh lemon juice
1 tbs finely shredded fresh
    mint leaves
1 red gem lettuce, leaves separated
½ bunch radishes, quartered

1 Line a tray with paper towel. Place the chickpeas on prepared tray and pat dry. Heat half the oil in a frying pan over medium heat. Add the chickpeas. Cook, stirring occasionally, for 6 minutes or until golden and crisp. Add the dukkah and cook, tossing, for 1 minute or until aromatic.
2 Meanwhile, place the beans and peas in a heatproof bowl. Cover with boiling water. Set aside for 2 minutes or until bright green and just tender. Drain. Refresh under cold running water.
3 Place the lemon juice, mint and remaining oil in a small bowl. Whisk to combine. Season. Arrange the lettuce on a serving platter. Top with the beans, peas, radish and chickpea mixture. Drizzle over the dressing to serve.

COOK'S NOTE

Don't have any dukkah? Coat the chickpeas in any combination of smoked paprika, garlic powder, ground cumin and coriander.

NUTRITION (PER SERVE)

CALS	FAT	SAT FAT	PROTEIN	CARBS
210	15.1g	1.8g	6.9g	9g

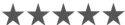

★★★★★

Fresh, crunchy and so much flavour, really enjoyed the zing. Will definitely be making again. A good base to add your own veg preferences as well. **NICS**

● EASY ● QUICK ○ MAKE AHEAD ● MEAT FREE ● FAMILY FRIENDLY

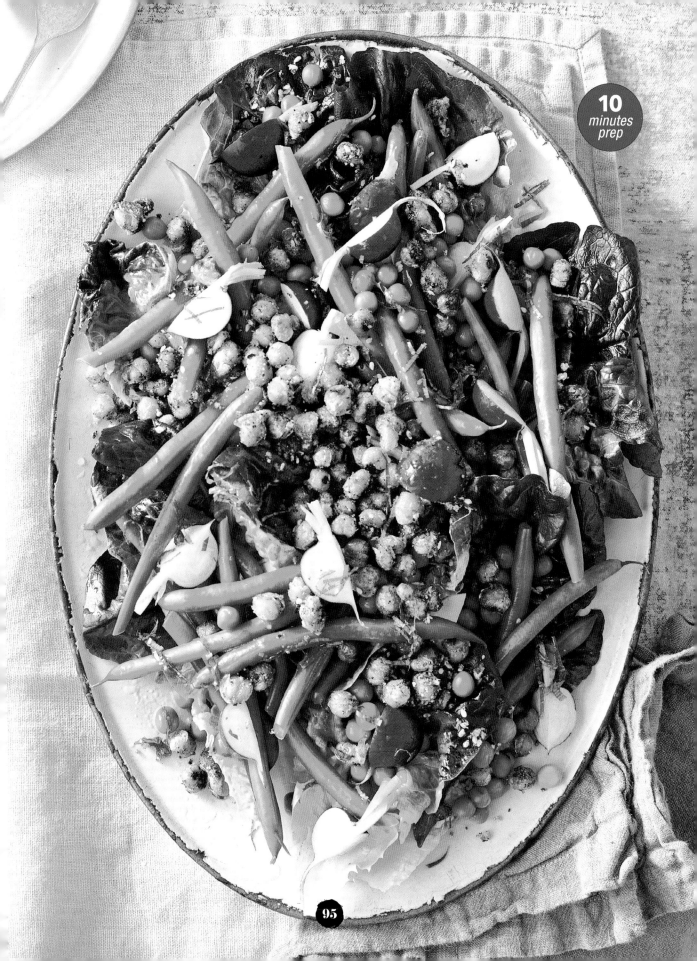

10
minutes
prep

Barbecued Peach
PANZANELLA

While you've got the barbecue fired up for your main, grill some peaches and bread, and you're halfway to building this fresh and fruity side.

SERVES 4 (as a side) **PREP** 10 mins **COOK** 10 mins

2 tbs white balsamic vinegar

1 tbs fresh lemon juice

70ml extra virgin olive oil

350g tomato medley mix, halved if large

2 cocktail truss tomatoes, coarsely chopped

1 small red onion, thinly sliced

1 small red capsicum, deseeded, finely chopped

3 fresh peaches, quartered

150g sliced sourdough bread

1 garlic clove, halved

130g Greek feta, crumbled

1½ cups firmly packed fresh herbs (such as basil and mint)

1 Combine the vinegar, lemon juice and 2½ tbs oil in a jar. Season well. Seal and shake to combine.

2 Combine the tomatoes, onion and capsicum in a large bowl. Add half the dressing. Toss to coat. Set aside for 5 minutes to develop the flavours.

3 Meanwhile, preheat a barbecue grill or chargrill on medium-high. Combine the peach and 2 tsp remaining oil in a bowl. Season. Grill the peach, turning, for 4 minutes or until charred and tender. Transfer to a plate. Brush the bread with the remaining oil. Grill the bread, turning, for 4 minutes or until charred. Rub with the cut side of the garlic. Coarsely tear the bread into large pieces.

4 Add the feta, herbs, peach and bread to the tomato mixture. Add the remaining dressing and gently toss to combine. Transfer to a serving plate, season and serve immediately.

COOK'S NOTE

This panzanella goes well with grilled lean chicken or salmon. Just cook at the same time as the peaches and bread.

NUTRITION (PER SERVE)

CALS	FAT	SAT FAT	PROTEIN	CARBS
441	24g	7g	14g	38g

★★★★★

*This looked so beautiful I gave it a whirl.
Fabulous flavour combo of sweet peaches and salty cheese.*

HARMONYPUFFIN

● EASY ● QUICK ○ MAKE AHEAD ● MEAT FREE ● FAMILY FRIENDLY

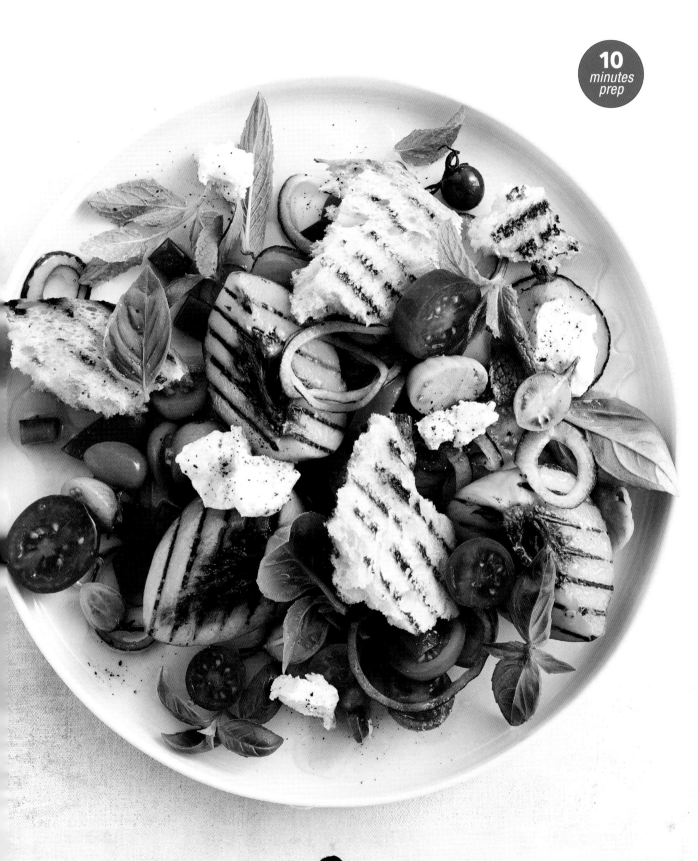

Sticky Grilled
FIG & BARLEY

The fig season is short, so make the most of it in sweet and savoury recipes. Here, the luscious fruit pairs beautifully with zesty orange dressing.

SERVES 4 (as a side) **PREP** 15 mins **COOK** 25 mins

- 165g (¾ cup) pearl barley, rinsed, drained
- 1 bunch asparagus, trimmed, halved lengthways
- ¼ tsp ground cumin
- 3 tsp honey
- 4 small figs, halved
- 60ml (¼ cup) fresh orange juice
- 1 tbs extra virgin olive oil
- 2 tsp balsamic vinegar
- 1cm piece fresh ginger, peeled, finely grated
- 2 tsp finely grated orange rind
- ½ small red onion, thinly sliced
- 60g mixed salad leaves
- ¼ cup fresh continental parsley leaves

1 Place the barley and 750ml (3 cups) water in a saucepan over high heat. Bring to the boil. Reduce heat to low and simmer for 25 minutes or until tender and liquid is almost absorbed. Drain and refresh under cold running water. Transfer to a large bowl.

2 Meanwhile, preheat a barbecue grill or chargrill pan to medium-high. Grill the asparagus, turning, for 2 minutes or until beginning to char. Transfer to a large plate. Combine the cumin and 2 tsp honey in a small bowl. Place the fig halves, cut-side up, on a large plate. Lightly sprinkle with the spice mixture. Grill the fig halves, cut-side down, for 1 minute or until beginning to char. Transfer to the plate.

3 Whisk together the orange juice, oil, vinegar, ginger, orange rind and remaining honey in a small bowl.

4 Add the asparagus, fig, onion, salad leaves and parsley to the barley. Pour over the dressing. Season and toss to combine. Transfer to a serving platter.

COOK'S NOTE

Pearl barley makes a great addition to salads. It has a chewy consistency and a nutty flavour. Find it in the soup aisle at the supermarket, near the lentils, beans and soup mix.

NUTRITION (PER SERVE)

CALS	FAT	SAT FAT	PROTEIN	CARBS
215	5.8g	0.7g	5.7g	31.2g

★★★★★

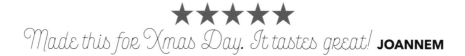

Made this for Xmas Day. It tastes great! **JOANNEM**

● EASY ○ QUICK ○ MAKE AHEAD ● MEAT FREE ● FAMILY FRIENDLY

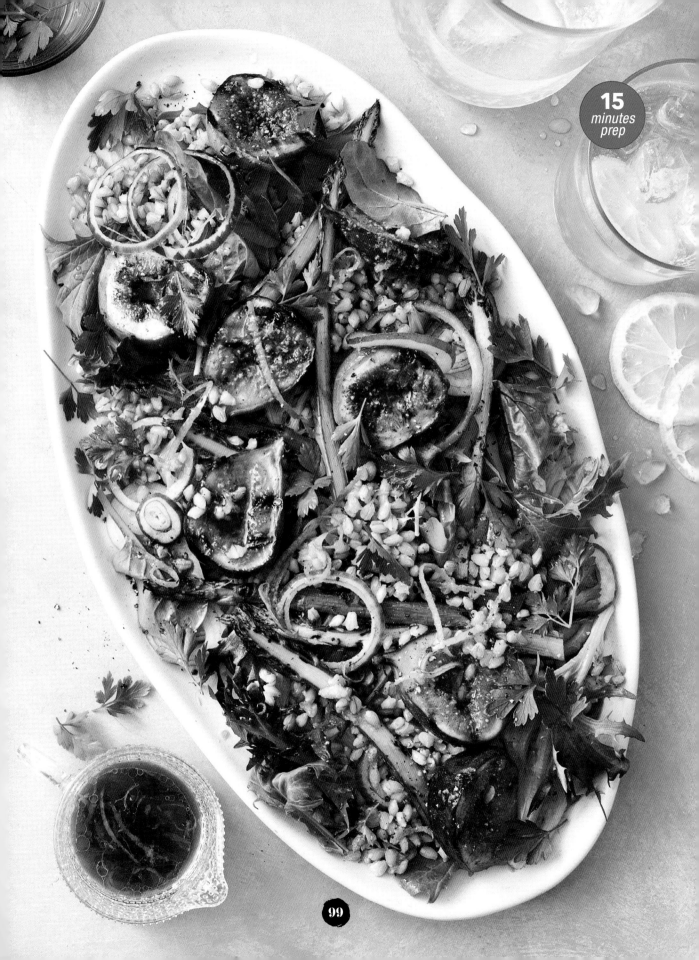

15
minutes
prep

Pan-Fried Feta GREEK SALAD

Tomatoes are heart-healthy, immunity-boosting goodies that deserve to be front and centre!

SERVES 4 (as a side) **PREP** 15 mins (+ 10 mins cooling) **COOK** 5 mins

200g block Greek feta, halved
   lengthways
2 tbs extra virgin olive oil
250g grape tomatoes, halved
200g yellow grape tomatoes, halved
1 green capsicum, deseeded,
   finely chopped
1 Lebanese cucumber,
   finely chopped
½ red onion, thinly sliced
80g (½ cup) pitted kalamata olives
¼ cup fresh oregano leaves
1 garlic clove, crushed
2 tbs fresh lemon juice

1 Pat dry the feta with paper towel. Heat 2 tsp oil in a non-stick frying pan over high heat. Add the feta and cook for 2 minutes on one side or until golden. Remove pan from heat. Set aside in the pan, without turning the feta, for 10 minutes to cool slightly.

2 Meanwhile, combine the tomatoes, capsicum, cucumber, onion, olives and half the oregano in a large bowl.

3 Whisk together the garlic, lemon juice and remaining oil in a small bowl until combined. Season. Drizzle the dressing over the salad. Transfer to a large serving plate. Place the feta, golden-side up, on top. Sprinkle with the remaining oregano to serve.

COOK'S NOTE

Serve this salad with pan-fried salmon fillets or grilled lamb skewers.

NUTRITION (PER SERVE)

CALS	FAT	SAT FAT	PROTEIN	CARBS
317	24.2g	9.6g	12.2g	8.6g

★★★★★

Getting real Med vibes from this plate. Loved the crispy feta on top.

DANI.BROUGHAM

● EASY ● QUICK ○ MAKE AHEAD ● MEAT FREE ● FAMILY FRIENDLY

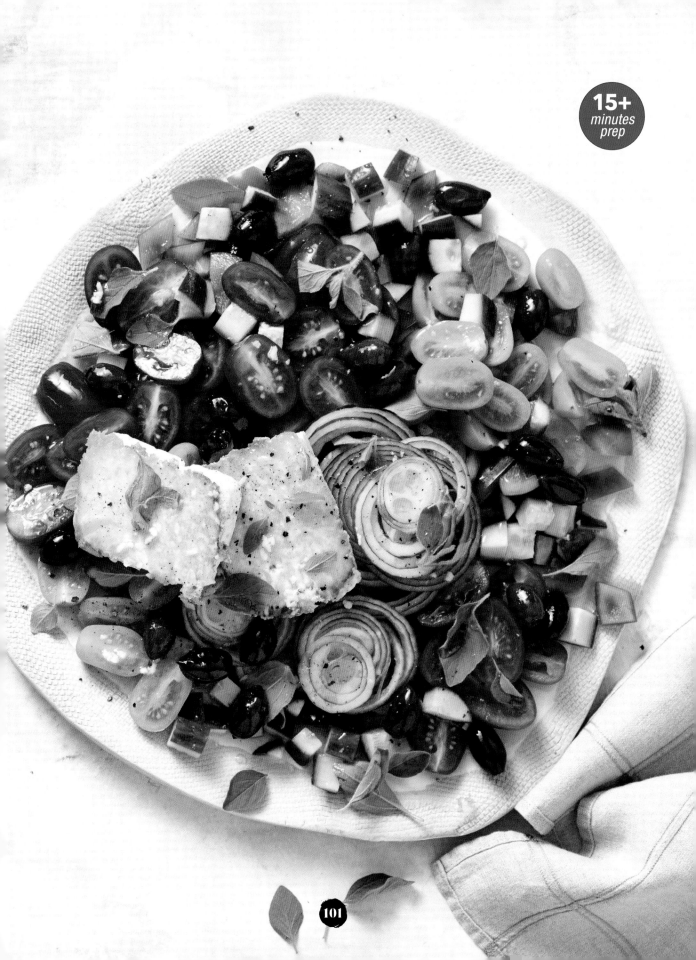

Brown Rice
BUTTERNUT SALAD

Roast pumpkin and cranberries star in this satisfying salad.
Serve it as a side and enjoy leftovers for tomorrow's lunch.

SERVES 6 (as a side) **PREP** 10 mins **COOK** 40 mins

500g butternut pumpkin, peeled,
   deseeded, cut into 2cm pieces
1 tbs extra virgin olive oil
200g (1 cup) brown rice
70g (½ cup) pecans, toasted,
   coarsely chopped
75g (½ cup) dried cranberries
3 green shallots, thinly sliced
1 cup fresh basil leaves
ORANGE DRESSING
2 tbs extra virgin olive oil
80ml (⅓ cup) fresh orange juice
1½ tbs white wine vinegar

1 Preheat oven to 200°C/180°C fan forced.
2 Arrange the pumpkin in a single layer in a baking dish.
Drizzle over the oil and roast for 40 minutes or until golden
and tender.
3 Meanwhile, cook the rice following packet directions.
4 To make the orange dressing, combine all the dressing
ingredients in a jar. Seal and shake until combined.
5 Combine the pumpkin, rice, pecans, cranberries and
dressing in a large bowl. Toss until combined. Season
then transfer to a serving platter. Sprinkle with the shallot
and basil to serve.

**COOK'S
NOTE**

Turn this side dish
into a main with
the addition of
shredded cooked
chicken, crumbled
feta or fried tofu.

NUTRITION (PER SERVE)

CALS	FAT	SAT FAT	PROTEIN	CARBS
364	19.2g	2.3g	5.7g	40.1g

★★★★★

Made this last night and my partner especially enjoyed it.
TEEDUB

● EASY ○ QUICK ● MAKE AHEAD ● MEAT FREE ● FAMILY FRIENDLY

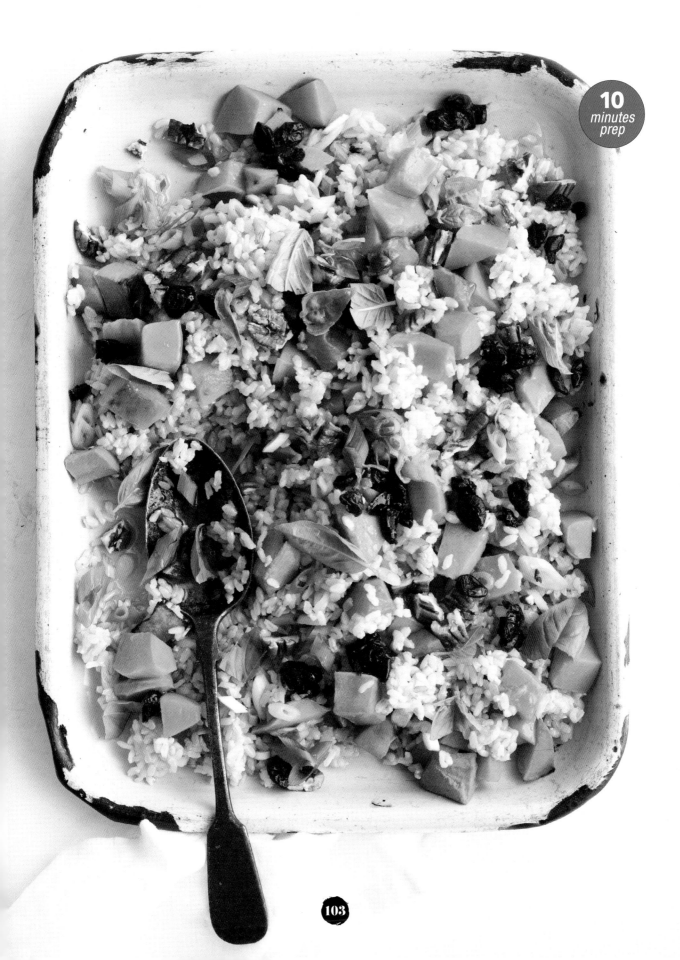

Broccolini & Bean
CHICKEN SALAD

With three vegies per serve and lean protein, this substantial salad is packed with good fats for heart health and will give you longer-lasting energy.

SERVES 4 **PREP** 20 mins **COOK** 10 mins

1½ tbs extra virgin olive oil
1 large chicken breast
150g green beans
1 bunch broccolini, trimmed, halved lengthways
400g can cannellini beans, rinsed, drained
3 green shallots, thinly sliced
1 avocado, sliced
4 radishes, sliced
60g baby rocket
2 tbs fresh lemon juice
1 tbs finely chopped fresh mint leaves, plus extra to serve
1 tbs finely chopped pistachio kernels
4 soft-boiled eggs, halved

1 Heat 2 tsp oil in a frying pan over medium-high heat. Cook the chicken for 4 minutes each side or until cooked through. Transfer to a plate. Cover loosely with foil. Set aside for 5 minutes to rest. Slice.
2 Meanwhile, cook the green beans and broccolini in a large saucepan of boiling water for 3 minutes or until bright green and tender. Drain. Refresh under cold running water. Transfer to a large serving bowl.
3 Add the cannellini beans, shallot, avocado, radish, rocket and chicken to the broccolini mixture. Toss gently.
4 Place the lemon juice, mint, pistachio and remaining oil in a small bowl. Season and stir to combine.
5 Top the salad with the egg and extra mint. Drizzle over the dressing to serve.

COOK'S NOTE

Use any vegies in season, such as asparagus, snow peas or zucchini. Replace radish with thinly sliced carrot, if not available. Serve with steamed brown rice or quinoa, if you like.

NUTRITION (PER SERVE)

CALS	FAT	SAT FAT	PROTEIN	CARBS
391	22.6g	4.7g	29.8g	11.1g

★★★★★

A super healthy, light meal that is now on the favourites list! Highly recommended. **EMMANUELG**

● EASY ● QUICK ○ MAKE AHEAD ○ MEAT FREE ● FAMILY FRIENDLY

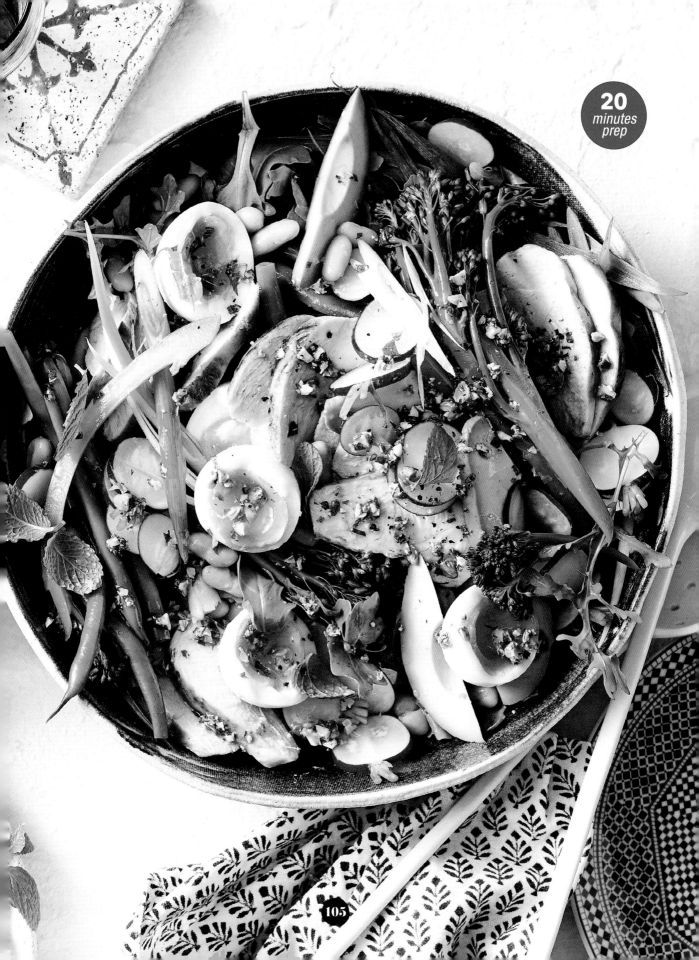

Broad Bean & Herb
SALMON QUINOA

Serve up this quick and easy smoked salmon salad for a healthy dose of veg and omega-3. Plus, it's pretty enough to make the cut when entertaining.

SERVES 4 **PREP** 15 mins **COOK** 15 mins

200g (1 cup) tri-colour quinoa,
  rinsed, drained
300g frozen broad beans (see note)
2 celery sticks, finely chopped
2 tbs finely chopped fresh chives
2 tbs finely chopped fresh dill,
  plus extra to serve
150g hot smoked salmon,
  skin removed, flesh flaked
75g Greek feta, crumbled
2 tbs sunflower seeds,
  lightly toasted
1 tsp lemon rind
1 tbs fresh lemon juice
1 tbs extra virgin olive oil
12 baby cos lettuce leaves
Lemon wedges, to serve

1 Place the quinoa and 435ml (1¾ cups) water in a saucepan and bring to the boil. Reduce heat to low, cover and simmer for 12-15 minutes or until the water is absorbed. Remove from heat and set aside to cool.
2 Meanwhile, blanch the broad beans in a saucepan of boiling water for about 2 minutes or until tender crisp. Refresh under cold running water. Drain. Peel off the skins.
3 Place the quinoa, broad beans, celery, chives, dill, salmon, feta, sunflower seeds and lemon rind in a large bowl. Season with pepper. Whisk together the lemon juice and oil in a small bowl then add to the quinoa mixture. Gently stir to combine.
4 Arrange the cos and quinoa mixture on a serving plate. Top with extra dill. Serve with lemon wedges to squeeze over.

COOK'S NOTE

Want to skip peeling broad beans? Swap for frozen peas to speed up the prep time even more.

NUTRITION (PER SERVE)

CALS	FAT	SAT FAT	PROTEIN	CARBS
388	16.3g	4.9g	23.9g	35g

★★★★★

Loved the crunch factor of all those greens and the ease of just throwing in smoked salmon. **VIOLAPARMESAN**

● EASY ● QUICK ○ MAKE AHEAD ○ MEAT FREE ● FAMILY FRIENDLY

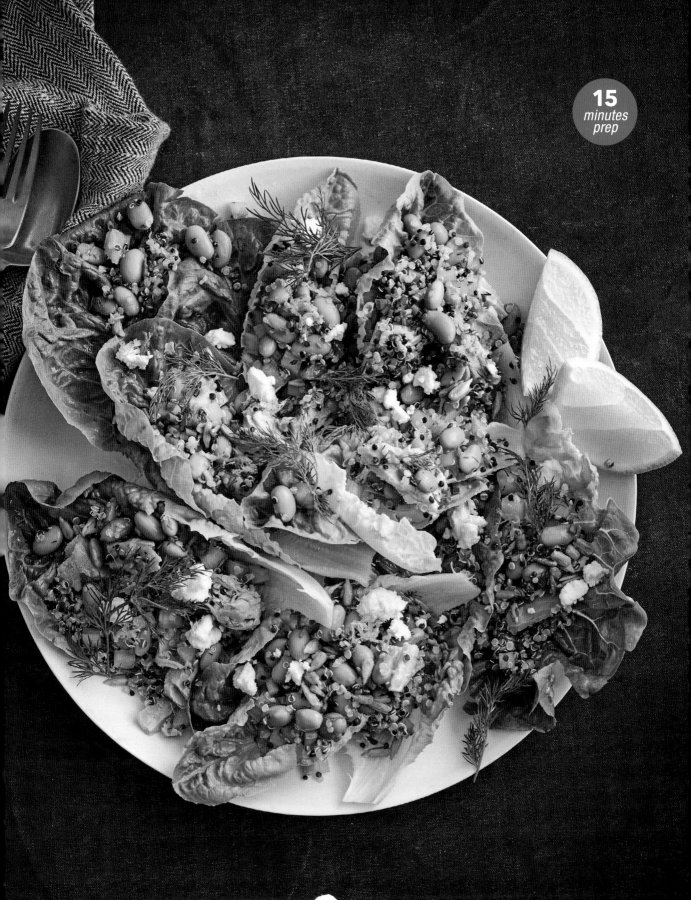

Pickles & Spring Vegie
FREEKEH

Packed with healthy greens, this delicious side stars freekeh, an ancient grain that is high in protein and fibre.

SERVES 4 (as a side) **PREP** 30 mins (+ 5 mins standing) **COOK** 35 mins

180g (1 cup) freekeh, rinsed, drained
1 bunch asparagus, trimmed
1 zucchini, very thinly sliced
1 yellow squash, very thinly sliced
2 tbs fresh lemon juice (see note)
1 tbs extra virgin olive oil,
   plus extra to drizzle
Pinch of dried chilli flakes
2 radishes, very thinly sliced
1 cup watercress sprigs
125g (½ cup) smooth ricotta
Thin strips of lemon rind, to serve

1 Place the freekeh and 750ml (3 cups) water in a saucepan over high heat. Bring to the boil. Reduce heat to low. Simmer, covered, for 35 minutes, adding the asparagus in the last 2 minutes of cooking, or until tender and liquid is absorbed. Set aside, covered, for 5 minutes.
2 Meanwhile, place the zucchini and squash in a bowl. Add the lemon juice, oil and chilli. Season. Stir to combine.
3 Spoon the freekeh and asparagus onto a large serving platter. Top with the pickled zucchini and squash, radish and watercress. Spoon over the pickling liquid. Dollop with the ricotta and drizzle over some extra oil. Sprinkle with lemon rind, season and serve.

COOK'S NOTE

Freekeh is a type of green wheat that has been roasted. Find it at selected supermarkets or health food shops. It can be cooked up to 1 day ahead and kept in the fridge. Cut the rind (for garnish) from the lemon before juicing – much easier this way!

NUTRITION (PER SERVE)

CALS	FAT	SAT FAT	PROTEIN	CARBS
318	10.1g	3.6g	11.8g	39.3g

★ ★ ★ ★ ★

I'd never had freekeh before, but it was easy to prepare. Great to add another grain to the repertoire.

BAKINGSELFIES

● **EASY**   ○ QUICK   ○ MAKE AHEAD   ● **MEAT FREE**   ○ FAMILY FRIENDLY

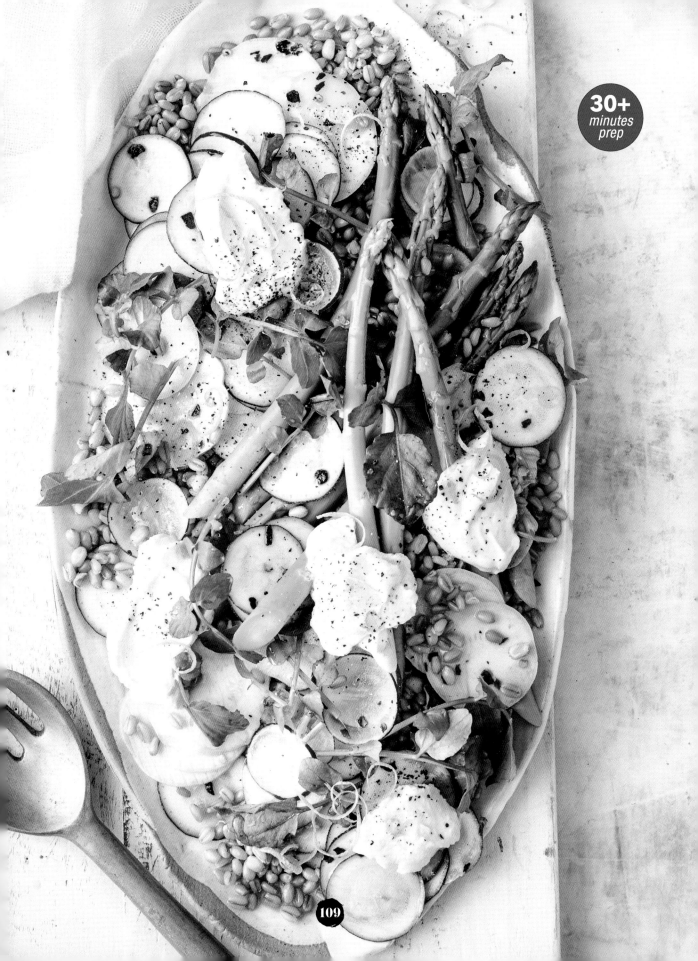

30+
minutes
prep

Whipped Basil Feta
GRILLED VEGIES

This colourful crowd-pleaser is like an antipasto plate in salad form! Grill your veg and prep the whipped feta ahead to make entertaining extra easy.

SERVES 6 (as a side) **PREP** 30 mins **COOK** 20 mins

2 red capsicums
2 small zucchini, thinly sliced lengthways
250g butternut pumpkin, unpeeled, thinly sliced
1 small eggplant, thinly sliced
2 tsp fresh thyme leaves
2 tbs garlic-infused extra virgin olive oil
200g cocktail truss tomatoes, cut into smaller bunches
175g mini capsicums
2 tbs pine nuts, coarsely chopped
1 tsp finely grated lemon rind
50g mixed salad leaves
WHIPPED BASIL FETA
200g Greek feta, crumbled
60ml (¼ cup) milk
1 tbs extra virgin olive oil
1 tbs fresh lemon juice (grate the rind for the salad before juicing)
2 tbs finely chopped fresh basil leaves

1 Quarter the red capsicums. Remove and discard the seeds and membrane. Place in a large bowl. Add the zucchini, pumpkin, eggplant and thyme. Drizzle over 1½ tbs garlic-infused oil. Toss to coat.
2 Preheat a barbecue grill or chargrill pan on high. Cook the red capsicum for 4 minutes each side or until tender and skin is blistered and blackened. Transfer to a sealable plastic bag and seal.
3 Transfer the zucchini, pumpkin and eggplant to grill. Cook the pumpkin for 3 minutes each side, and zucchini and eggplant for 2 minutes each side or until charred and tender. Transfer to a bowl. Add the tomato and mini capsicums to grill. Cook for 2 minutes or until beginning to char and collapse. Set aside to cool slightly.
4 Meanwhile, make the whipped basil feta. Place the feta, milk, oil and lemon juice in a small food processor. Process until smooth, scraping down side (do not over-process). Transfer to a bowl. Add the basil. Season with pepper and stir to combine.
5 Heat the remaining garlic-infused oil in a small frying pan over low heat. Add the pine nuts. Cook, stirring, for 3 minutes or until just golden. Add the lemon rind. Cook for 1 minute.
6 Peel and discard the skin from the red capsicum. Add to the vegetable mixture along with the salad leaves. Toss to combine. Arrange the mixture on a large serving plate. Top with the tomato, mini capsicums, whipped feta and pine nut mixture.

NUTRITION (PER SERVE)

CALS	FAT	SAT FAT	PROTEIN	CARBS
296	21.5g	6.9g	11g	11.7g

○ EASY ○ QUICK ● MAKE AHEAD ● MEAT FREE ● FAMILY FRIENDLY

★★★★★
This is a beautiful salad. It both looks and tastes good.
It is easy to prepare a bit earlier and then assemble when needed.

WENDYMAV

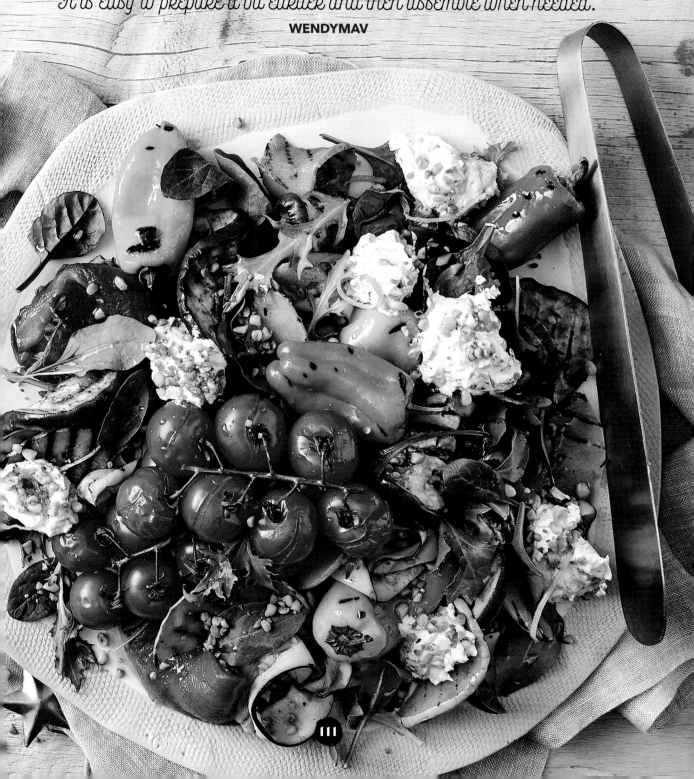

Chermoula-Grilled
CALAMARI SALAD

This spicy seafood grill is big on nutrition and flavour. Calamari is a high-quality source of protein and the omega-3 fatty acid DHA, essential for brain function.

SERVES 4 **PREP** 20 mins (+ 1 hour marinating) **COOK** 10 mins

1 long fresh red chilli, deseeded, chopped
1 cup fresh continental parsley leaves
1 cup fresh coriander leaves
2 garlic cloves, crushed
2 tsp ground cumin
2 tsp ground paprika
60ml (¼ cup) fresh lemon juice
1 tbs extra virgin olive oil
500g calamari, scored, cut into 7cm pieces,
1 red onion, finely chopped
400g can chickpeas, rinsed, drained
200g green beans, halved, steamed
150g chargrilled red capsicum (not in oil), sliced
Lemon wedges, to serve

1 Place the chilli and half each of the parsley, coriander, garlic, cumin and paprika in a food processor. Process until finely chopped. Add 2 tbs lemon juice and 2 tsp oil. Process until a paste forms.
2 Place the calamari in a bowl. Add the chilli mixture and mix well. Cover and place in the fridge for 1 hour to marinate.
3 Heat the remaining oil in a saucepan over medium-high heat. Cook the onion, stirring, for 3-4 minutes or until light golden. Add the remaining garlic, cumin and paprika. Stir for 1 minute or until aromatic. Add the chickpeas, remaining 1 tbs lemon juice and 60ml (¼ cup) water. Simmer for 1 minute. Mash with a fork.
4 Heat a chargrill pan over high heat. Spray the calamari lightly with extra virgin olive oil. Cook for 1-2 minutes each side or until just cooked through.
5 Spoon the chickpea mixture onto a serving plate. Top with the beans, capsicum, calamari and remaining herbs. Serve with lemon wedges to squeeze over.

COOK'S NOTE

Don't overcrowd the chargrill pan with calamari, as the temperature can drop and it will stew rather than sear. If your pan is small, cook the calamari in batches. Serve with wholemeal pita bread, if you like.

NUTRITION (PER SERVE)

CALS	FAT	SAT FAT	PROTEIN	CARBS
279	9g	1g	28g	14g

★★★★★
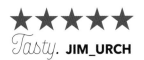
Tasty. **JIM_URCH**

● **EASY** ○ QUICK ○ MAKE AHEAD ○ MEAT FREE ○ FAMILY FRIENDLY

20+
minutes
prep

★★★★★

Easy and simple. Something different. **SNELLY**

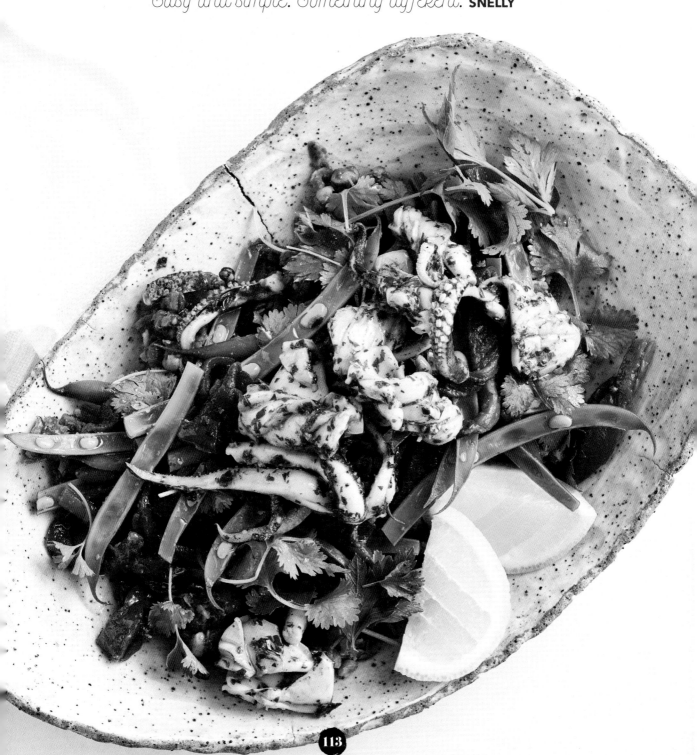

113

Orange Spiced
CAULI & LAMB

Add nuts and seeds to your salad for an easy nutrient booster. Here, they're roasted until crispy for that real crunch factor.

SERVES 4 **PREP** 20 mins (+ 15 mins standing) **COOK** 45 mins

180g (1 cup) freekeh, rinsed, drained
35g (¼ cup) pecan halves
1 tbs sunflower seeds
1 tbs pepitas
60ml (¼ cup) honey
3 oranges
1 tsp ground cumin
800g cauliflower, cut into florets
1 red onion, cut into thin wedges
2 tbs extra virgin olive oil
400g lean lamb leg steaks
1 tbs apple cider vinegar
½ cup fresh mint leaves
½ cup fresh continental
  parsley leaves

1 Preheat oven to 200°C/180°C fan forced. Line a large baking tray with baking paper.
2 Place the freekeh and 750ml (3 cups) water in a saucepan over high heat. Bring to the boil. Reduce heat to low. Simmer, covered, for 35 minutes or until tender and liquid is absorbed. Set aside, covered, for 5 minutes. Combine the pecans, sunflower seeds, pepitas and 1 tbs honey in a bowl. Season.
3 Meanwhile, finely grate the rind from 2 oranges (you'll need 1 tbs in total). Reserve the oranges. Place the cumin and 2 tsp orange rind in a large bowl. Add the cauliflower and onion. Toss to coat. Transfer to prepared tray. Spray with extra virgin olive oil. Roast for 15 minutes.
4 Spoon level teaspoonfuls of the seed mixture onto tray. Roast for a further 5 minutes or until the cauliflower is tender and the seed mixture is golden and crisp.
5 Combine the remaining 2 tsp orange rind and 1 tbs of remaining honey in a small bowl. Heat half the oil in a large, non-stick frying pan over medium-high heat. Cook the lamb, brushing with the honey mixture, for 2 minutes each side for medium or until cooked to your liking. Transfer to a plate. Cover loosely with foil. Set aside for 10 minutes to rest. Slice.
6 Juice the remaining orange (you'll need 2 tbs juice). Place the juice, vinegar, remaining honey and remaining oil in a small bowl. Stir until the honey dissolves. Season. Peel and slice the reserved oranges. Place the freekeh, cauliflower mixture, orange slices, mint, parsley, orange juice mixture and lamb in a serving bowl. Toss to combine then serve.

NUTRITION (PER SERVE)

CALS	FAT	SAT FAT	PROTEIN	CARBS
653	26.3g	4.7g	34.8g	66.7g

● EASY ○ QUICK ○ MAKE AHEAD ○ MEAT FREE ● FAMILY FRIENDLY

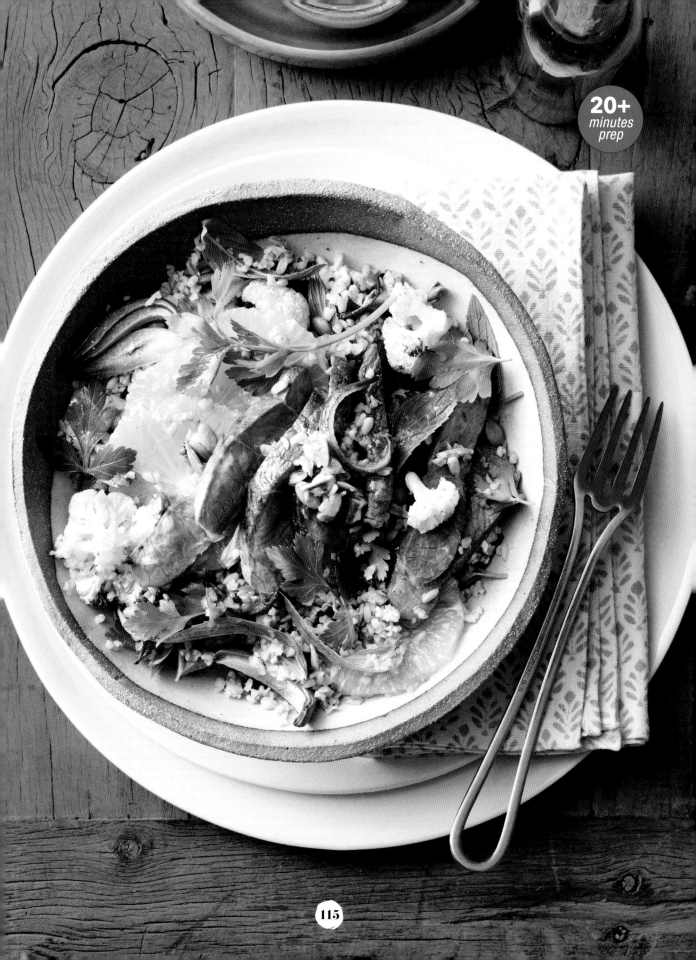

Grilled Asparagus
TOMATO SALAD

Bookmark this one for when tomatoes are at their peak. The combo of herbs and preserved lemon is the secret to adding loads of flavour.

SERVES 4 (as a side) **PREP** 15 mins (+ cooling) **COOK** 10 mins

4 slices wholemeal sourdough bread
2 bunches asparagus, trimmed
1½ tbs extra virgin olive oil
1 garlic clove, halved
350g tomato medley mix,
   halved, quartered if large
200g grape tomatoes, halved
½ cup fresh basil leaves
½ cup fresh continental
   parsley leaves
1 tbs baby capers, rinsed,
   drained, chopped
1 tbs white balsamic vinegar
1 preserved lemon quarters,
   peel only, rinsed, finely chopped
   (see note)

1 Preheat a barbecue grill or chargrill pan on high. Brush the bread slices and asparagus with 1 tbs oil.
2 Grill the bread for 2 minutes each side or until lightly charred. Grill the asparagus for 1-2 minutes each side or until just tender. Transfer the bread and asparagus to a plate. Rub the bread with the cut side of the garlic and set aside to cool slightly.
3 Tear the bread into bite-size pieces. Combine the bread, asparagus, tomatoes, basil, parsley and capers in a large bowl. Season.
4 Whisk together the vinegar, preserved lemon and remaining oil. Add to the salad and gently toss to combine. Transfer to a serving plate to serve.

COOK'S NOTE

To prepare the preserved lemon, discard the pulpy flesh but don't remove the pith as you would with a fresh lemon or orange.

NUTRITION (PER SERVE)

CALS	FAT	SAT FAT	PROTEIN	CARBS
196	8.1g	1.2g	7.9g	19.1g

★★★★★

I love tomatoes and this looked so amazing as part of a spread.

DRPRETTY

● EASY ● QUICK ○ MAKE AHEAD ● MEAT FREE ○ FAMILY FRIENDLY

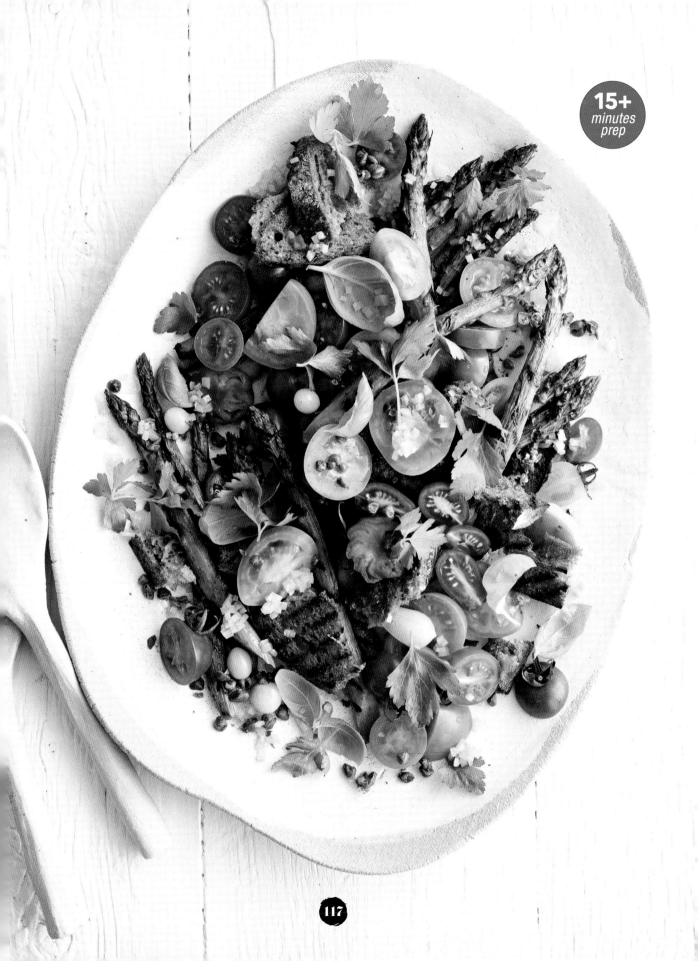

15+
minutes
prep

Zesty Salmon
VEGIE COUSCOUS

It's super easy to lift a plate of vegies and seafood to new, fresh heights with just the lightest touch. This is a lovely light lunch or starter.

SERVES 4 (as a starter) **PREP** 10 mins (+ cooling) **COOK** 15 mins

150g skinless salmon fillet
2 bunches asparagus, trimmed
1 large zucchini, peeled into ribbons
400g can chickpeas, rinsed, drained
½ small red onion, thinly sliced
½ cup fresh continental
  parsley leaves
150g wholemeal couscous
150ml boiling water
90g (⅓ cup) low-fat Greek-style
  yoghurt
1 tbs fresh lemon juice
2 tbs chopped fresh chives
Lemon wedges, to serve

1 Preheat oven to 180°C/160°C fan forced. Line a baking tray with baking paper.
2 Place the salmon on prepared tray. Bake for 8-10 minutes or until cooked through. Set aside to cool slightly then flake into pieces.
3 Preheat a barbecue grill or chargrill pan on high. Lightly spray the asparagus and zucchini with extra virgin olive oil. Grill the asparagus and zucchini for 2 minutes each side or until charred and tender crisp. Transfer to a plate. Halve the asparagus lengthways. Combine the salmon, asparagus, zucchini, chickpeas, onion and parsley in a bowl.
4 Place the couscous in a heatproof bowl then pour over the boiling water. Cover and set aside for 3-4 minutes or until all the liquid is absorbed. Use a fork to separate the grains.
5 Whisk the yoghurt, lemon juice and chives in a bowl. Divide the couscous and salmon mixture among serving plates. Drizzle over the dressing and serve with lemon wedges to squeeze over.

COOK'S NOTE

If you prefer, cook the salmon on the chargrill instead. Skip step 1 and 2, and grill the salmon after the vegies in step 3. It will take about 3 minutes each side.

NUTRITION (PER SERVE)

CALS	FAT	SAT FAT	PROTEIN	CARBS
295	4g	1g	21g	41g

★ ★ ★ ★ ★

I will definitely be making it again. Made great leftovers. **ALIHAT**

● EASY ● QUICK ○ MAKE AHEAD ○ MEAT FREE ● FAMILY FRIENDLY

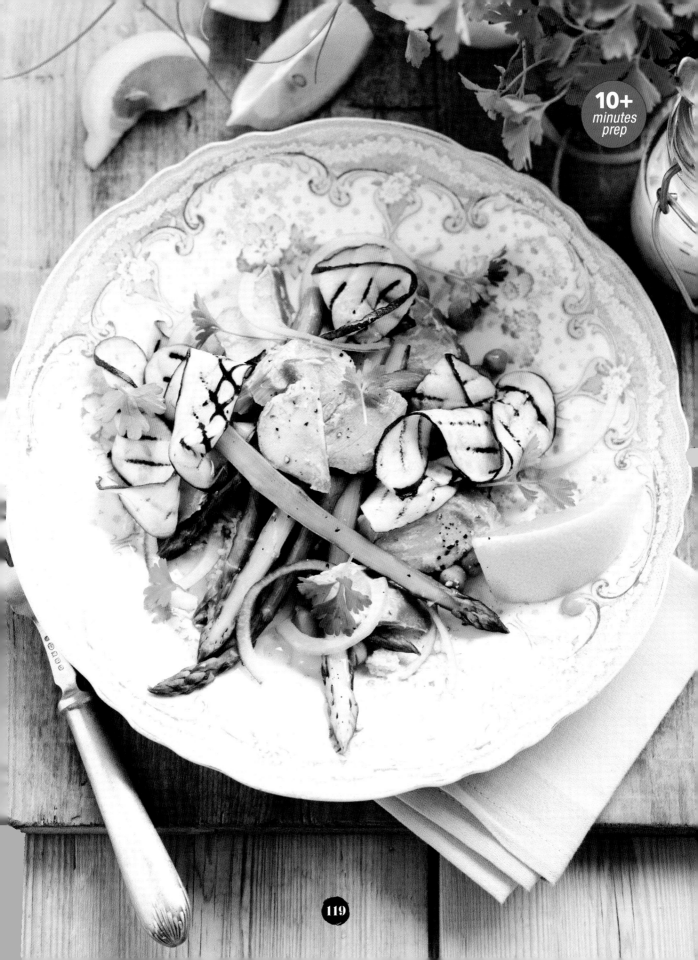

10+
minutes
prep

Chickpea & Pomegranate
HONEY CARROTS

Serve a crowd this nutrient-packed platter, rich in betacarotene for healthy immunity, iron and vitamin C to boost iron absorption.

SERVES 6 (as a side) **PREP** 15 mins **COOK** 30 mins

2 tbs extra virgin olive oil
2 tsp honey
2 tsp finely grated lemon rind
3 bunches baby carrots,
    scrubbed, trimmed
400g can chickpeas, rinsed, drained
1½ tsp whole coriander seeds
1½ tbs white balsamic vinegar
½ bunch watercress, leaves picked
45g (¼ cup) toasted hazelnuts,
    coarsely chopped
1 tbs pomegranate arils
Red-vein sorrel leaves or
    baby spinach, to serve

1 Preheat oven to 200°C/180°C fan forced. Line a large baking tray with baking paper.
2 Combine 1 tbs oil, 1 tsp honey and 1 tsp lemon rind in a small bowl. Place the carrots on prepared tray, drizzle over the honey mixture and toss to combine. Bake for 20 minutes. Add the chickpeas to the tray and bake for a further 10 minutes or until the carrots are golden and tender.
3 Meanwhile, toast the coriander seeds in a small frying pan over medium heat for 1-2 minutes or until aromatic. Use the back of a spoon to lightly crush. Place the crushed coriander seeds, vinegar and remaining oil, honey and lemon rind in a small bowl and stir to combine. Season.
4 Arrange the watercress, carrots and chickpeas on a large serving platter. Scatter over the hazelnut, pomegranate and sorrel or spinach. Drizzle over the dressing to serve.

COOK'S NOTE

Use small regular carrots, if you prefer. Cut them lengthways into quarters.

NUTRITION (PER SERVE)

CALS	FAT	SAT FAT	PROTEIN	CARBS
233	10.5g	1.2g	10.6g	14.4g

★★★★★

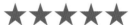

This was my contribution to Christmas lunch. Everyone loved it!
WAFFLEISO

● EASY ○ QUICK ○ MAKE AHEAD ● MEAT FREE ● FAMILY FRIENDLY

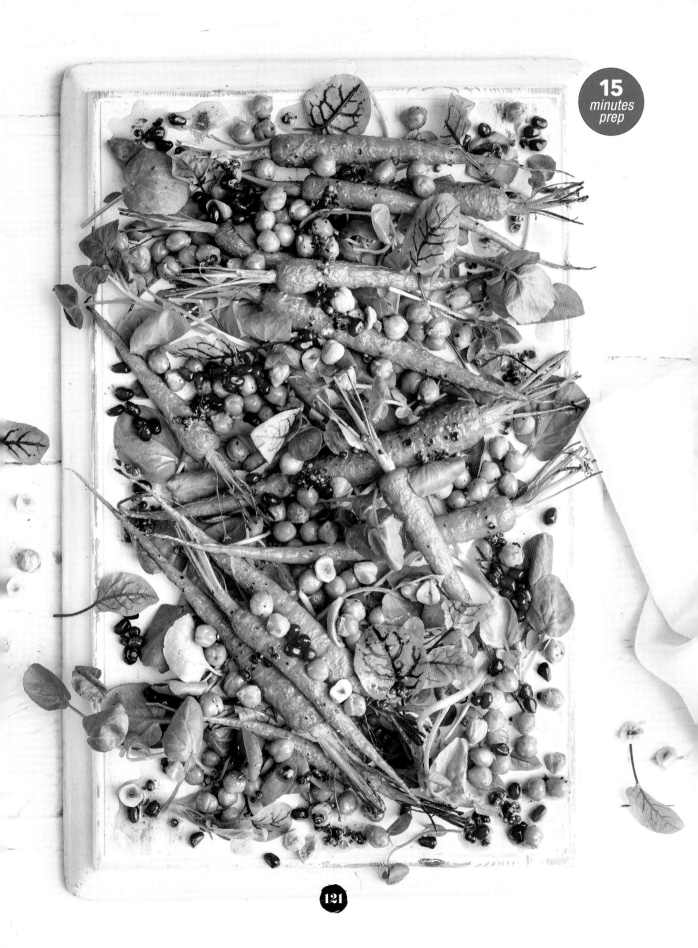

Currant & Dill
BROWN RICE

Turn microwave brown rice into a full blown meal with zucchini, soft-boiled eggs and a quick cumin, currant and citrus dressing.

SERVES 4 **PREP** 10 mins **COOK** 5 mins

2 x 250g pkt microwave brown rice
4 eggs
1 small lemon, rind finely grated, juiced
2 tbs extra virgin olive oil
2 tbs dried currants
1 tsp ground cumin
1 bunch fresh dill
1 large zucchini, finely chopped
4 green shallots, thinly sliced
2 tbs toasted pine nuts

1 Cook the rice following packet directions. Transfer to a large bowl. Set aside to cool slightly.

2 Meanwhile, bring a small saucepan of water to the boil over high heat. Add the eggs. Reduce heat to medium and cook for 4 minutes for soft yolks or until cooked to your liking. Refresh in a bowl of iced water. Peel the eggs.

3 Place the lemon rind and juice, oil, currants and cumin in a small bowl. Season and stir to combine.

4 Chop half the dill. Add the chopped dill, remaining dill sprigs, zucchini, shallot and half the pine nuts and dressing to the rice. Toss to combine. Transfer to a serving bowl. Carefully tear the eggs in half and arrange on top of the rice salad. Drizzle over the remaining dressing and sprinkle with the remaining pine nuts. Season and serve.

NUTRITION (PER SERVE)

CALS	FAT	SAT FAT	PROTEIN	CARBS
443	22g	3g	13g	47g

COOK'S NOTE

Serve with steamed green beans, if you like. Looking for other ways to use up pine nuts? Toss over a tray of roast veg in the last 10 minutes of cooking or swirl through brown butter with a squeeze of lemon to scatter over fish.

★★★★★

Really tasty! I added cherry tomatoes and cranberries. Lots of flavour.

MADIH

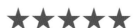

● EASY ● QUICK ○ MAKE AHEAD ● MEAT FREE ● FAMILY FRIENDLY

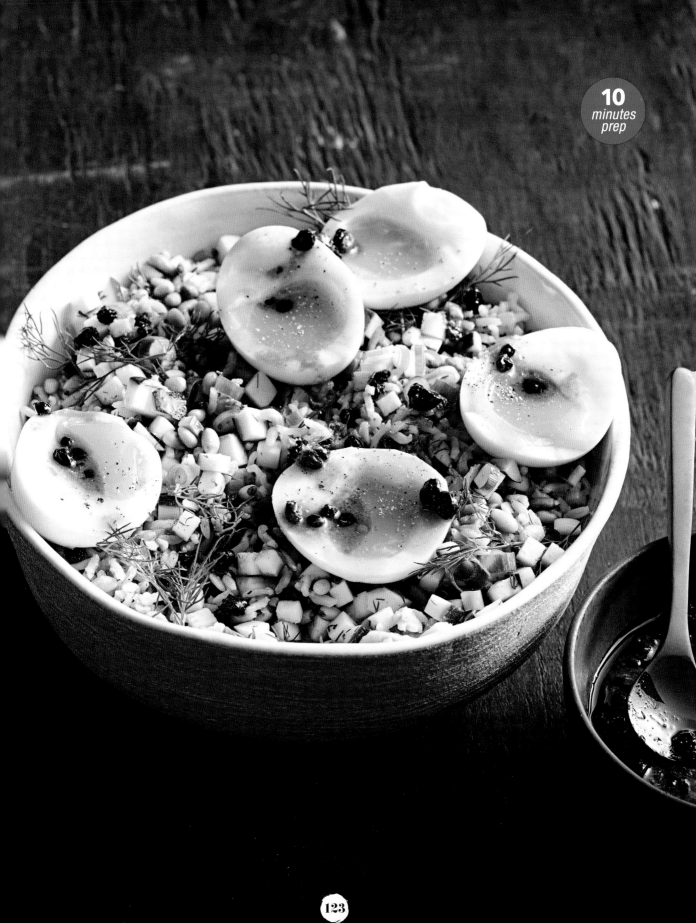

Spicy & Smoky Calamari
POTATO SALAD

Spruce up your healthy salad repertoire with sensational seafood and legumes. Squid and chickpeas are protein powerhouses.

SERVES 4 **PREP** 15 mins (+ 1 hour marinating & cooling) **COOK** 15 mins

2 tbs fresh lemon juice
1½ tbs extra virgin olive oil
1½ tsp harissa paste
2 tsp smoked paprika
500g calamari, scored,
   cut into 3cm pieces
400g kipfler potatoes, scrubbed
   (see note)
1 red onion, thinly sliced
400g can chickpeas, rinsed, drained
1 large chargrilled red capsicum
   (not in oil), sliced
200g green beans, steamed,
   halved lengthways
100g baby rocket

1 Combine 1 tbs lemon juice, 2 tsp oil, 1 tsp harissa and 1 tsp paprika in a shallow dish. Add the calamari and turn to coat. Cover and place in the fridge for 1 hour to marinate.
2 Combine the remaining lemon juice and harissa in a small bowl.
3 Cook the potato in a steamer basket over a saucepan of boiling water for 12-15 minutes or until tender. Drain and set aside to cool slightly then cut into 1.5cm-thick slices.
4 Meanwhile, heat 2 tsp remaining oil in a large non-stick frying pan over high heat. Cook the calamari for 1-2 minutes each side or until golden and just cooked through. Transfer to a plate. Return the pan to medium heat. Add the onion and remaining oil. Cook, stirring, for 3-4 minutes or until almost softened. Add the chickpeas and remaining paprika. Cook for 2 minutes. Add the capsicum and cook for 1 minute or until heated through. Pour in the lemon juice mixture. Season and toss until combined.
5 Combine the warm chickpea mixture, potato, beans and rocket in a large bowl then divide among serving bowls. Top with the calamari and drizzle over any pan juices. Serve immediately.

COOK'S NOTE

Kipfler is a variety of potato which are long tubers rather than round. They are great for salads or for roasting. Use baby coliban (chat) potatoes instead, if not available.

NUTRITION (PER SERVE)

CALS	FAT	SAT FAT	PROTEIN	CARBS
340	10.6g	1.7g	30.2g	26.4g

● EASY ○ QUICK ○ MAKE AHEAD ○ MEAT FREE ○ FAMILY FRIENDLY

15+
minutes
prep

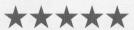
★ ★ ★ ★ ★

Using the same ingredients for the squid marinade as the dressing made it extra easy and less bits to buy.

FANCY FOODIE

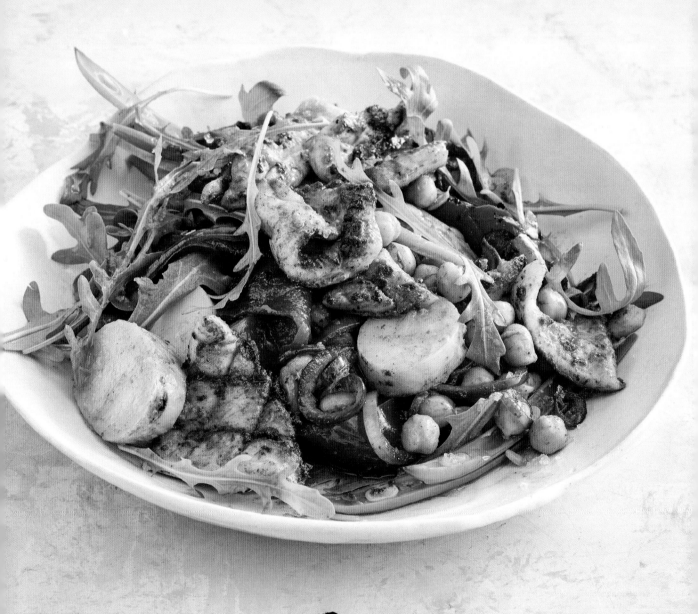

Rainbow & Fruity
POWER PLATE

Team colourful nutritious vegies, such as broccoli and tomato, with chickpeas and freekeh. Top it off with blueberries for extra antioxidants.

SERVES 4 **PREP** 20 mins **COOK** 15 mins

400g can chickpeas, rinsed, drained

70g (⅓ cup) tri-colour quinoa, rinsed, drained

60g (⅓ cup) freekeh, rinsed, drained

1 head (about 350g) broccoli, trimmed, cut into florets

145g (1 cup) frozen peeled broad beans (see note)

200g tomato medley mix, halved

4 radishes, thinly sliced

½ cup fresh mint leaves, plus extra to serve

2 tbs pepitas

1 tbs apple cider vinegar

1 tbs extra virgin olive oil

1 tbs honey

70g (½ cup) fresh blueberries

1 Preheat oven to 200°C/180°C fan forced. Grease a baking tray and line with baking paper.

2 Spread the chickpeas over prepared tray. Spray lightly with extra virgin olive oil. Bake for 15 minutes or until golden and crisp.

3 Meanwhile, cook the quinoa and freekeh in a large saucepan of boiling water for 12 minutes or until just tender. Drain. Refresh under cold running water.

4 Place the broccoli and broad beans in a steamer basket over a saucepan of simmering water. Cover and steam for 3-4 minutes or until just tender. Drain. Refresh under cold running water.

5 Combine the grain mixture, broccoli, broad beans, tomato, radish, mint and pepitas in a large bowl. Season.

6 Whisk together the vinegar, oil and honey in a small bowl. Add the dressing to the salad and gently toss to combine. Divide among serving plates. Top with the roasted chickpeas, blueberries and extra leaves just before serving.

COOK'S NOTE

If you can't get peeled broad beans, simply slip them out of their skins after refreshing.

NUTRITION (PER SERVE)

CALS	FAT	SAT FAT	PROTEIN	CARBS
339	10.6g	1.5g	17.4g	36g

★★★★★

The recipes are always so easy, taste delicious and are very economical and healthy. **CRISSI71**

● EASY ○ QUICK ○ MAKE AHEAD ● MEAT FREE ● FAMILY FRIENDLY

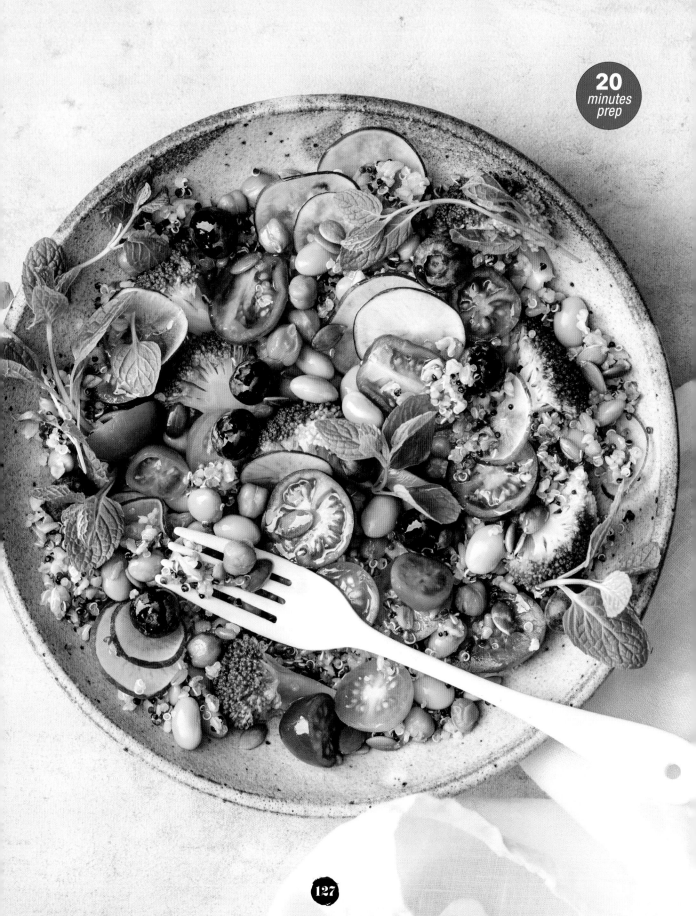

Roast Salmon & Cauliflower
SPICED BURGHUL

Nourishing burghul with roast vegetables, salmon and a garlicky yoghurt dressing makes a hearty meal-in-a-salad.

SERVES 4 **PREP** 15 mins (+ 30 mins soaking) **COOK** 35 mins

135g (¾ cup) burghul
½ (about 550g) cauliflower,
   cut into small florets
1 red onion, cut into wedges
2 tbs extra virgin olive oil,
   plus extra to serve
1 tsp ground sumac, plus extra
   to sprinkle
1 tsp ground cumin
1 tsp ground coriander
2 large skinless salmon fillets
1 lemon, rind finely grated, halved
2 garlic cloves, crushed
130g (½ cup) Greek-style yoghurt
1 tbs tahini
1 cup fresh mint leaves
1 cup fresh coriander leaves

1 Preheat oven to 210°C/190°C fan forced. Line 2 baking trays with baking paper.
2 Place the burghul in a bowl and cover with cold water. Set aside for 30 minutes to soak. Drain. Spread over a clean tea towel. Bring together the tea towel and squeeze to remove excess liquid. Transfer to a bowl.
3 Meanwhile, place the cauliflower and onion on 1 prepared tray. Drizzle over 1½ tbs oil. Season. Combine the sumac, cumin and coriander in a bowl. Sprinkle the vegetables with 1 teaspoonful of the spice mixture. Roast, stirring once, for 25 minutes or until golden.
4 Place the salmon on the remaining prepared tray. Season. Add the lemon rind, half the garlic and remaining oil to the remaining spice mixture then drizzle over the salmon. Roast the salmon for the last 12 minutes of vegetable cooking time or until cooked to your liking. Set aside for 3 minutes to rest. Coarsely flake.
5 Juice 1 lemon half. Combine the yoghurt, tahini, 1 tbs water, 1½ tbs lemon juice and remaining garlic in a bowl. Season.
6 Chop three-quarters of the herbs. Add the roast vegetables and chopped herbs to the burghul. Toss to combine. Divide among serving plates. Top with the salmon. Drizzle over the dressing and extra oil. Sprinkle with the remaining herbs and extra sumac. Serve with the remaining lemon half to squeeze over.

NUTRITION (PER SERVE)

CALS	FAT	SAT FAT	PROTEIN	CARBS
565	30g	7g	39g	31g

★★★★★

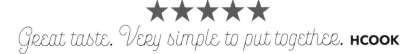

Great taste. Very simple to put together. **HCOOK**

○ EASY   ○ QUICK   ● MAKE AHEAD   ● MEAT FREE   ● FAMILY FRIENDLY

15+
minutes
prep

★★★★★
Loved this. Super yummy. Will definitely make again and again.
ALEXANDRA

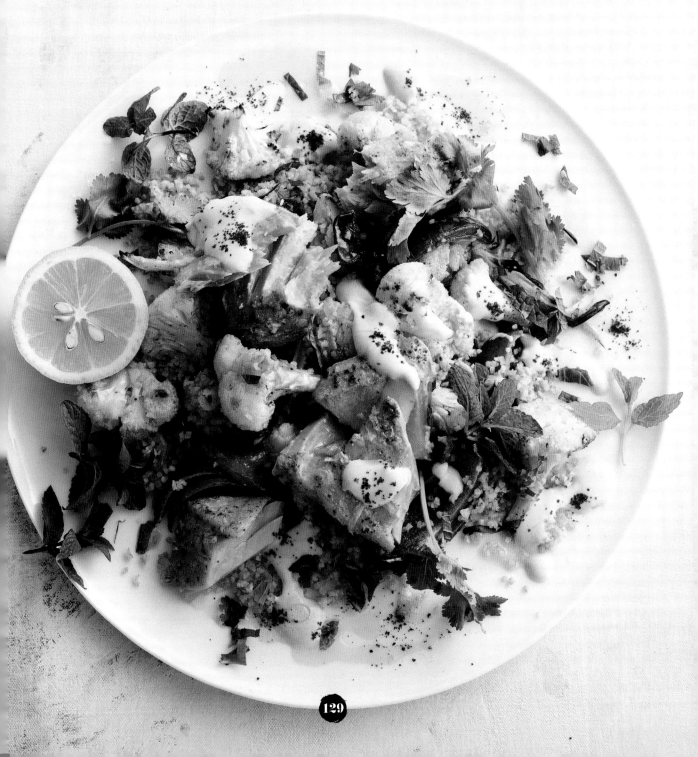

Warm Balsamic
BEETS & LENTILS

There are plenty of shortcuts to make this simple side oh-so easy! Microwave rice, canned lentils and cooked beetroot mean it's ready in 20 minutes.

SERVES 4 (as a side) **PREP** 10 mins **COOK** 10 mins

250g pkt microwave brown rice

400g can brown lentils, rinsed, drained

2 tsp extra virgin olive oil

250g pkt whole cooked beetroot, cut into wedges

2 tbs balsamic vinegar

2 tsp honey

90g (⅓ cup) Greek-style yoghurt

1 tbs chopped fresh dill

1 tbs fresh lemon juice

½ small red onion, thinly sliced

½ cup fresh continental parsley leaves

35g (⅓ cup) flaked almonds, toasted

1 Heat the rice following packet directions. Transfer to a heatproof bowl. Add the lentils. Season and stir to combine.
2 Meanwhile, heat the oil in a large frying pan over medium-high heat. Add the beetroot. Cook, turning occasionally, for 4 minutes or until heated through. Add the vinegar and honey. Cook, turning occasionally, for 3 minutes or until the liquid is almost evaporated.
3 Combine the yoghurt, dill and lemon juice in a small bowl. Season.
4 Transfer the rice mixture to a serving platter. Top with the beetroot, onion, parsley and almonds. Dollop with the yoghurt dressing to serve.

COOK'S NOTE

Add a large can of tuna in olive oil to turn this beauty into lunch.

NUTRITION (PER SERVE)

CALS	FAT	SAT FAT	PROTEIN	CARBS
376	14g	2.4g	13.4g	44.5g

★★★★★

Lovely healthy salad. All the flavours complement each other well.

MAMBA87

● EASY ● QUICK ○ MAKE AHEAD ● MEAT FREE ● FAMILY FRIENDLY

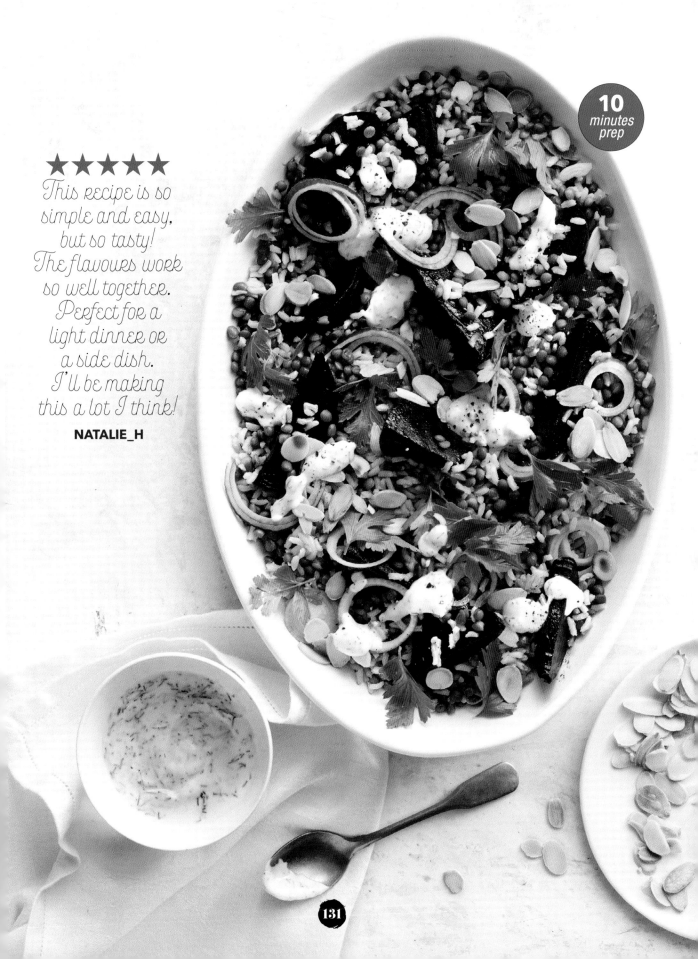

★★★★★

This recipe is so simple and easy, but so tasty! The flavours work so well together. Perfect for a light dinner or a side dish. I'll be making this a lot I think!

NATALIE_H

10 minutes prep

Orange Poppyseed
SUPER CRUNCH

Julienne your way to a crispy, colourful combo with raw carrot, beetroot, brussels sprouts and more!

SERVES 4 (as a side) **PREP** 15 mins **COOK** 5 mins

4 eggs
1 large carrot, peeled, cut into
  long thin strips (see note)
1 large beetroot, peeled, cut into
  thin strips (see note)
6 brussels sprouts, thinly sliced
1 small fennel bulb, thinly sliced
¼ small head broccoli, thinly
  sliced lengthways
2 tbs finely chopped fresh chives
DRESSING
2 tbs fresh orange juice
2 tbs extra virgin olive oil
1 tbs fresh lemon juice
1 garlic clove, smashed
2 tsp poppyseeds

1 To make the dressing, combine all the dressing ingredients in a jar. Season. Seal and shake until combined.
2 Place the eggs in a small saucepan and cover with boiling water. Bring to the boil, stirring occasionally, and cook for 3 minutes. Drain. Refresh under cold running water. Peel and slice in half.
3 Combine the carrot, beetroot, sprouts, fennel and broccoli in a large bowl. Drizzle over the dressing and toss to coat. Divide among serving bowls. Top with the egg and chives.

NUTRITION (PER SERVE)

CALS	FAT	SAT FAT	PROTEIN	CARBS
202	14.2g	2.8g	8.2g	12.2g

COOK'S NOTE

Use a julienne peeler to cut the carrot and beetroot into long thin strips. If you don't have a julienne peeler, thinly slice then cut into thin strips.

★★★★★

Raw all the way is fine by me!
FOODSLED

● EASY   ● QUICK   ○ MAKE AHEAD   ● MEAT FREE   ● FAMILY FRIENDLY

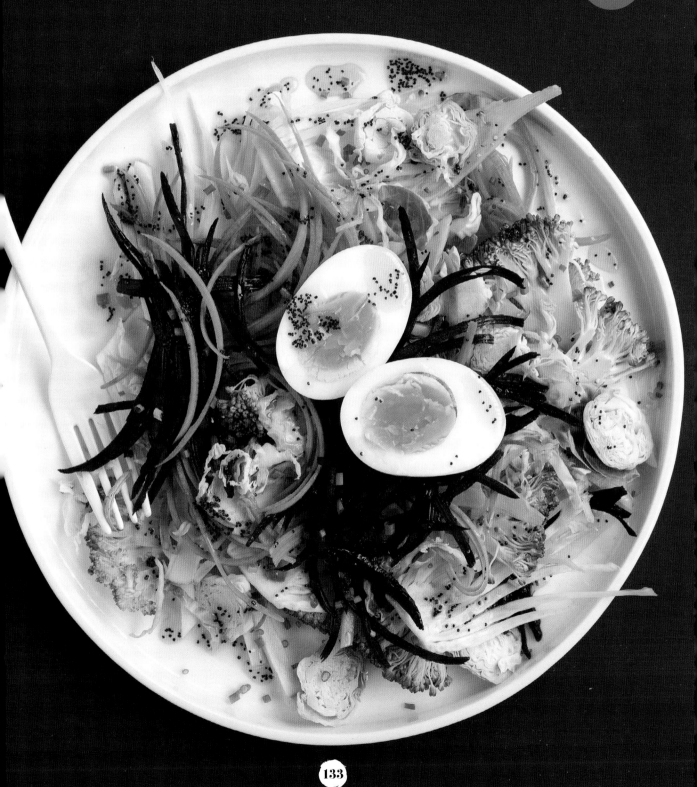

Roast Chickpea
BROCCOLI BOWL

Deliciously seasoned roast chickpeas and crispy chips made from wholegrain wraps take this veg-full salad to a whole new level. Prep is a breeze too.

SERVES 4 **PREP** 20 mins (+ cooling) **COOK** 35 mins

1 tsp ground cumin

1 tbs extra virgin olive oil

3 tsp honey

400g can no-added-salt chickpeas, rinsed, drained

300g broccoli, cut into florets

1 tbs tahini

1 tbs fresh lemon juice

2 wholegrain wraps

250g cherry tomatoes, halved

1 large Lebanese cucumber, halved, coarsely chopped

½ cup fresh mint leaves, coarsely chopped

½ cup fresh continental parsley leaves, coarsely chopped

40g Greek feta, crumbled

1 Preheat oven to 200°C/180°C fan forced. Line 2 baking trays with baking paper.

2 Combine the cumin, 2 tsp oil and 2 tsp honey in a large bowl. Add the chickpeas and toss until combined. Spread the chickpeas over 1 prepared tray. Roast, stirring occasionally, for 25 minutes or until golden and crisp.

3 Meanwhile, cook the broccoli in a steamer basket over a saucepan of boiling water for 3 minutes or until bright green and tender crisp. Drain. Refresh under cold running water. Coarsely chop. Whisk together the tahini, lemon juice and remaining honey and oil in a small bowl. Add 2-3 tsp water until a dressing-like consistency.

4 Cut the wraps into wedges. Place on remaining prepared tray. Lightly spray with extra virgin olive oil. Bake for 8 minutes or until golden. Set aside to cool.

5 Combine the broccoli, tomato, cucumber, mint and parsley in a large bowl. Season. Toss through the wrap wedges and feta. Spoon onto a large serving platter. Top with the chickpeas and tahini dressing. Serve immediately.

COOK'S NOTE

These roast chickpeas are also great as an arvo snack or as part of an antipasto platter. They'll keep in an airtight container for up to a day.

NUTRITION (PER SERVE)

CALS	FAT	SAT FAT	PROTEIN	CARBS
279	13g	3.4g	13g	18.7g

● EASY ○ QUICK ○ MAKE AHEAD ● MEAT FREE ● FAMILY FRIENDLY

20+
minutes
prep

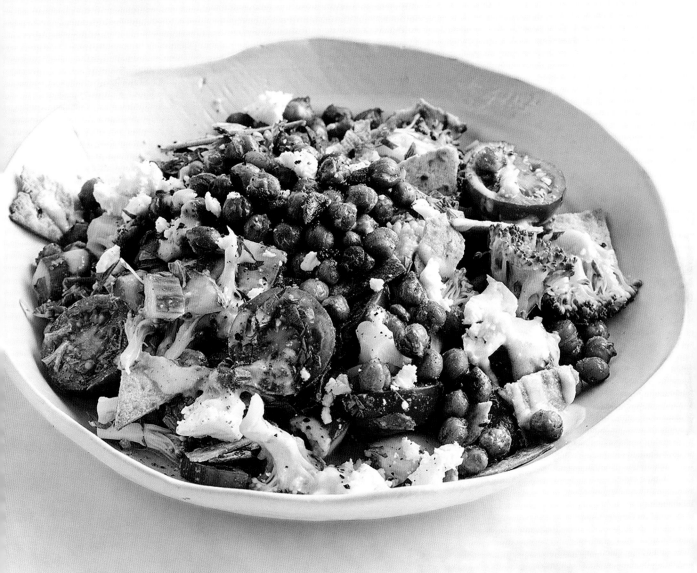

★★★★★
Very nice, simple meal.
ALISONJAYM

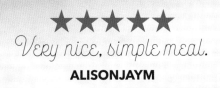

135

Prawn & Pea
MIXED GRAINS

Pimp your prawns with quinoa and buckwheat – they're nutritious wholegrains, rich in dietary fibre and plant protein.

SERVES 4 **PREP** 20 mins (+ 5 mins pickling) **COOK** 15 mins

75g (⅓ cup) buckwheat,
  rinsed, drained
70g (⅓ cup) tri-colour quinoa,
  rinsed, drained
Pinch of table salt
Pinch of caster sugar
2 tbs white balsamic vinegar
1 red onion, thinly sliced
200g snow peas
150g (1 cup) frozen green peas
1 tbs extra virgin olive oil
200g grape tomatoes, halved
1 cup fresh mint leaves
1 cup fresh continental
  parsley leaves
350g peeled cooked prawns,
  tails intact
2 tbs chopped pistachio kernels
Ground sumac and lemon wedges,
  to serve

1 Cook the buckwheat and quinoa in a large saucepan of boiling water for 10-12 minutes or until al dente. Drain. Refresh under cold running water.
2 Combine the salt, sugar and 1 tbs vinegar in a small bowl. Add the onion and stir until coated. Set aside for 5 minutes to pickle.
3 Meanwhile, steam the snow peas and peas in a steamer over a saucepan of simmering water until just tender. Drain. Refresh under cold running water. Shred the snow peas.
4 Whisk together the oil and remaining vinegar in a small bowl.
5 Combine the quinoa mixture, snow peas, peas, tomato, mint and parsley in a large bowl then divide among serving plates. Top with the prawns, pickled onion and pistachio. Drizzle over the oil mixture and sprinkle with sumac. Serve with lemon wedges to squeeze over.

COOK'S NOTE

Sumac is a berry that has been dried and ground. It has a citrussy flavour, so you can replace with a squeeze of lemon juice, if you don't have any sumac.

NUTRITION (PER SERVE)

CALS	FAT	SAT FAT	PROTEIN	CARBS
378	8g	1.5g	32.9g	31.5g

★ ★ ★ ★ ★

I'm using this quick pickle on all my salads now!
DANI.BROUGHAM

● **EASY** ○ QUICK ○ MAKE AHEAD ○ MEAT FREE ○ FAMILY FRIENDLY

20+
minutes
prep

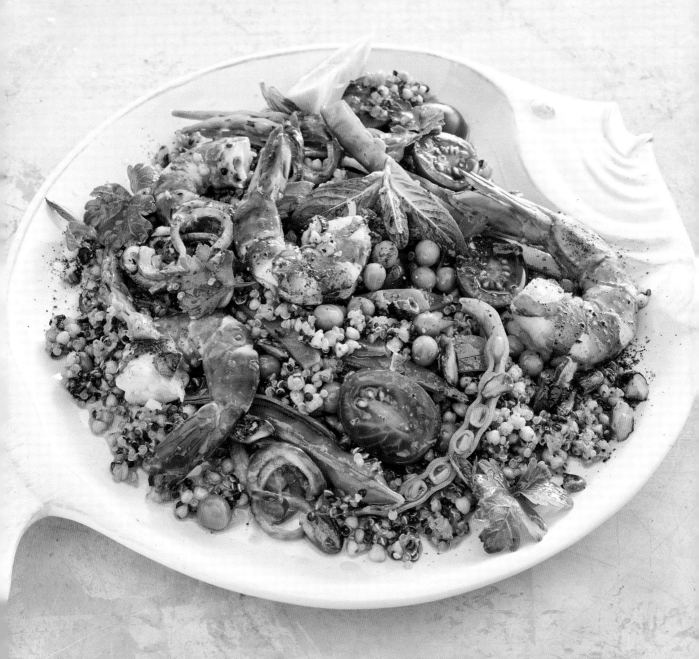

Quick Green Beans
TUNA & BEETS

Got only 15 minutes to spare? You've got enough time to make a nutritious and delicious salad that'll fill you up until dinner.

SERVES 4 **PREP** 10 mins **COOK** 5 mins

300g green beans, halved lengthways
400g whole cooked baby beetroot, cut into wedges
425g can tuna in olive oil, drained, flaked
120g mixed salad leaves
80g Greek feta, crumbled
2 tbs white balsamic vinegar
2 tbs fresh lemon juice
1 tbs extra virgin olive oil
1 tbs hemp seeds

1 Cook the green beans in a steamer basket over a saucepan of boiling water for 3 minutes or until bright green and tender crisp. Drain. Refresh under cold running water.
2 Combine the green beans, beetroot, tuna, salad leaves and feta in a serving bowl.
3 Whisk together the vinegar, lemon juice and oil in a jug. Drizzle the dressing over the salad. Divide among serving plates. Scatter over the hemp seeds and serve immediately.

COOK'S NOTE

Serve this salad with steamed wholemeal couscous or wholegrain sourdough bread, if you like.

NUTRITION (PER SERVE)

CALS	FAT	SAT FAT	PROTEIN	CARBS
267	9.9g	3.6g	26g	14.5g

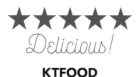

★★★★★
Delicious!
KTFOOD

● EASY ● QUICK ○ MAKE AHEAD ○ MEAT FREE ● FAMILY FRIENDLY

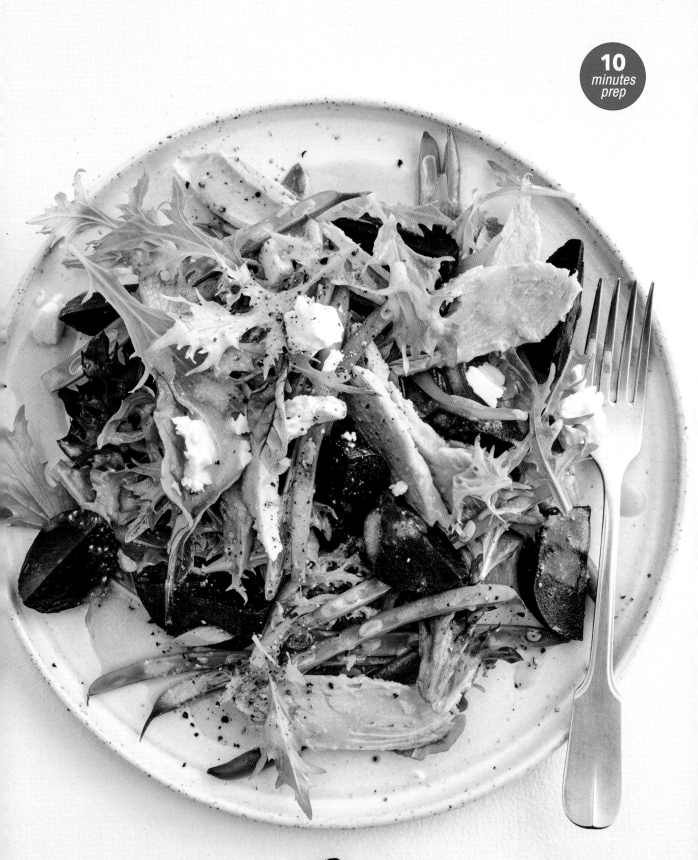

Honey & Cumin
ROAST VEGIES

Roasting the vegetables with orange juice and honey creates delicious caramelisation in this satisfying buckwheat salad.

SERVES 4 **PREP** 15 mins **COOK** 35 mins

2 bunches baby rainbow carrots, scrubbed, trimmed
2 red capsicums, deseeded, coarsely chopped
1 red onion, cut into wedges
2 tbs extra virgin olive oil
60ml (¼ cup) fresh orange juice
1 tsp cumin seeds
2 tsp finely grated fresh ginger
1 garlic clove, crushed
1½ tbs honey
200g buckwheat, rinsed, drained, dried
1½ tbs red wine vinegar
1 cup fresh coriander, firmly packed
1 cup firmly packed fresh continental parsley leaves
100g reduced-fat Greek feta, crumbled
40g baby rocket
45g (¼ cup) roasted almonds, coarsely chopped

1 Preheat oven to 200°C/180°C fan forced. Line 2 baking trays with baking paper.
2 Spread the carrots, capsicum and onion over prepared trays. Drizzle over half the oil. Season. Roast for 15 minutes.
3 Whisk together the orange juice, cumin, ginger, garlic and 1 tbs honey in a bowl. Drizzle over the vegetables. Roast, turning halfway, for a further 20 minutes or until tender.
4 Meanwhile, heat a non-stick frying pan over medium heat. Add the buckwheat and cook, stirring, for 2 minutes or until toasted. Set aside for 5 minutes to cool. Bring a saucepan of water to the boil over high heat. Add the buckwheat to the pan. Reduce heat to medium-low and simmer for 15 minutes or until al dente. Drain. Refresh under cold running water. Spread over a tray lined with paper towel to dry.
5 Whisk together the vinegar and remaining oil and honey in a large bowl. Season. Add the buckwheat, herbs, feta, rocket and roast vegetables. Toss to combine then transfer to a serving platter. Top with the almonds.

COOK'S NOTE

Cook the buckwheat and roast the vegetables up to two days in advance. Store in separate airtight containers in the fridge. Bring to room temperature before combining.

NUTRITION (PER SERVE)

CALS	FAT	SAT FAT	PROTEIN	CARBS
464	21g	5g	18g	52g

● EASY ○ QUICK ● MAKE AHEAD ● MEAT FREE ● FAMILY FRIENDLY

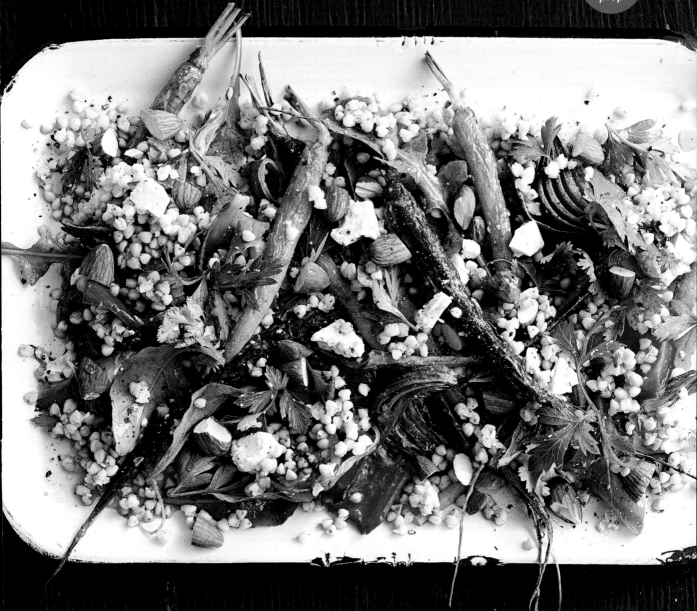

★ ★ ★ ★ ★

Love this recipe in autumn. Flavours are amazing! Easy to swap rainbow carrots for regular carrots to save $ too. We boost it with chicken tenderloins and finish it off with a drizzle of pomegranate molasses. **ALYSE-GRACE**

Green Goddess SMOKED SALMON

Salmon is rich in good fats and vitamin A (for vision and immunity) and D (for healthy bones). Drizzle over green goddess – the ultimate herby hero!

SERVES 4 **PREP** 15 mins (+ 5 mins pickling) **COOK** 20 mins

105g (½ cup) French-style green lentils, rinsed, drained

2 baby fennel bulbs, thinly sliced, some fronds reserved

130g (½ cup) Greek-style yoghurt

2 tbs chopped fresh continental parsley, plus extra leaves to serve

2 tbs chopped fresh chives

1 tbs chopped fresh tarragon leaves

1 tbs baby capers, rinsed, drained

1 tsp finely grated lemon rind

½ red onion, thinly sliced

1 tbs fresh lemon juice

Pinch of caster sugar

60g baby spinach

½ avocado, sliced

180g sliced salt-reduced smoked salmon

1 Cook the lentils in a large saucepan of boiling water for 20 minutes or until tender. Drain.

2 Meanwhile, preheat a barbecue grill or chargrill pan on high. Spray the fennel slices with extra virgin olive oil. Grill for 2 minutes each side or until tender.

3 Place the yoghurt, parsley, chives, tarragon, capers and lemon rind in a food processor. Season with pepper then process until smooth.

4 Place the onion, lemon juice and sugar in a bowl. Season with salt. Set aside for 5 minutes to pickle. Drain.

5 Combine the lentils, fennel, pickled onion, spinach and avocado in a large bowl. Divide among serving plates. Top with the salmon. Sprinkle with the reserved fennel fronds and extra parsley. Drizzle over the green goddess dressing. Season and serve.

COOK'S NOTE

Double the dressing and keep in the fridge for up to 4 days. Serve on other salads, spread over sandwiches or use as a dip. Serve this salad with wholegrain sourdough bread, if you like.

NUTRITION (PER SERVE)

CALS	FAT	SAT FAT	PROTEIN	CARBS
296	13g	3g	20g	20g

★★★★★

It was seriously delicious! I used salmon steaks instead, but smoked salmon would be great too. **MEG.DEM**

● **EASY** ○ QUICK ○ MAKE AHEAD ○ MEAT FREE ○ FAMILY FRIENDLY

★ ★ ★ ★ ★
Great lunch. **WENDY0407**

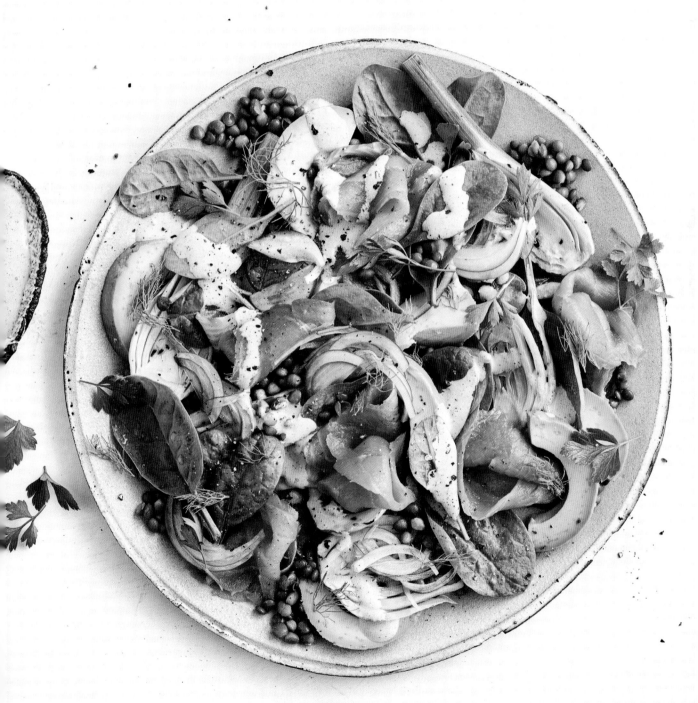

Cypriot
GRAIN SALAD

With so many textures and flavours, this vibrant burghul salad is packed full of ancient grains, nuts, seeds and dried fruits, with a zingy caper dressing.

SERVES 6 (as a side) **PREP** 10 mins (+ 20 mins soaking)

170g (1 cup) burghul, rinsed, drained
400g can no-added salt lentils, rinsed, drained
1 small red onion, finely chopped
1 cup chopped fresh coriander leaves
1 cup chopped fresh continental parsley leaves
80g (½ cup) seed mix (such as sunflower seeds, pepitas and pine nuts), toasted
75g (½ cup) dried cranberries, coarsely chopped
50g (¼ cup) drained capers, rinsed, coarsely chopped
45g (¼ cup) currants
35g (⅓ cup) flaked almonds, toasted
60ml (¼ cup) fresh lemon juice
60ml (¼ cup) extra virgin olive oil

1 Place the burghul in a heatproof bowl. Cover with boiling water. Set aside for 20 minutes or until tender. Drain. Transfer to a large serving bowl.
2 Add the remaining ingredients to the bowl. Season and gently toss until combined.

NUTRITION (PER SERVE)

CALS	FAT	SAT FAT	PROTEIN	CARBS
386	20.2g	2.8g	11.4g	44.2g

COOK'S NOTE

Serve as a side with any grilled chicken, fish or meat, or crumble over some feta for a vego meal.

★★★★★

OMG this is the best salad! It's constantly in my fridge and a firm family favourite. I use quinoa instead of burghul as I'm coeliac. It's so good to have a grainy salad I can eat! **KATHSTA**

● EASY ● QUICK ● MAKE AHEAD ● MEAT FREE ● FAMILY FRIENDLY

10+
minutes
prep

★ ★ ★ ★ ★
*Used tri-colour quinoa, but otherwise kept to recipe.
Definitely will be a next time.* **WMR309**

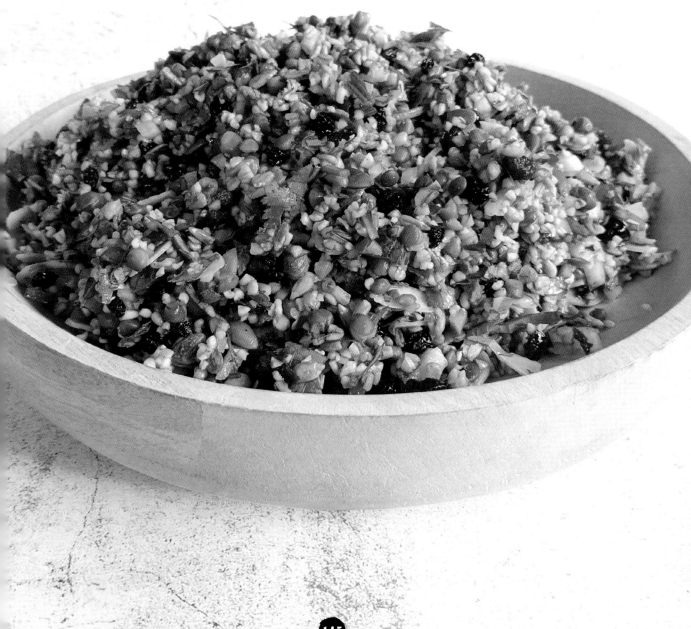

Yoghurt & Chickpea
SPICY ROASTIES

With broccoli, chickpeas, yoghurt and a creamy jalapeño dressing, this easy plate of roast vegetables is brimming with superfood goodness.

SERVES 4 (as a side) **PREP** 20 mins **COOK** 25 mins

½ tsp ground coriander

½ tsp ground cumin

2 bunches baby carrots, scrubbed, trimmed

1 red capsicum, deseeded, sliced

1 head (about 350g) broccoli, trimmed, cut into florets

400g can chickpeas, rinsed, drained

130g (½ cup) Greek-style yoghurt

1 fresh jalapeño chilli, deseeded, finely chopped

2 tbs chopped fresh coriander leaves

1 tbs fresh lemon juice

1 tbs warm water

75g baby spinach

1 Preheat oven to 200°C/180°C fan forced. Line 2 baking trays with baking paper.

2 Combine the ground coriander and cumin in a small bowl. Place the carrots and capsicum on 1 prepared tray. Place the broccoli and chickpeas on remaining prepared tray. Sprinkle the vegetable mixture evenly with the spice mixture. Spray with extra virgin olive oil. Roast the carrots and capsicum for 25 minutes and the broccoli and chickpeas for 12 minutes or until golden and tender.

3 Meanwhile, combine the yoghurt, chilli, fresh coriander, lemon juice and warm water in a bowl.

4 Place the roasted vegetables, chickpeas and spinach in a large bowl and gently toss to combine. Divide among serving plates and drizzle over the yoghurt dressing.

COOK'S NOTE

Roast the vegies and make the dressing up to 1 day ahead.

NUTRITION (PER SERVE)

CALS	FAT	SAT FAT	PROTEIN	CARBS
168	4g	1g	11g	17g

★★★★★

Yummy. Nice for a light lunch. The dressing sets it off.

DIHEN

● EASY ○ QUICK ● MAKE AHEAD ● MEAT FREE ○ FAMILY FRIENDLY

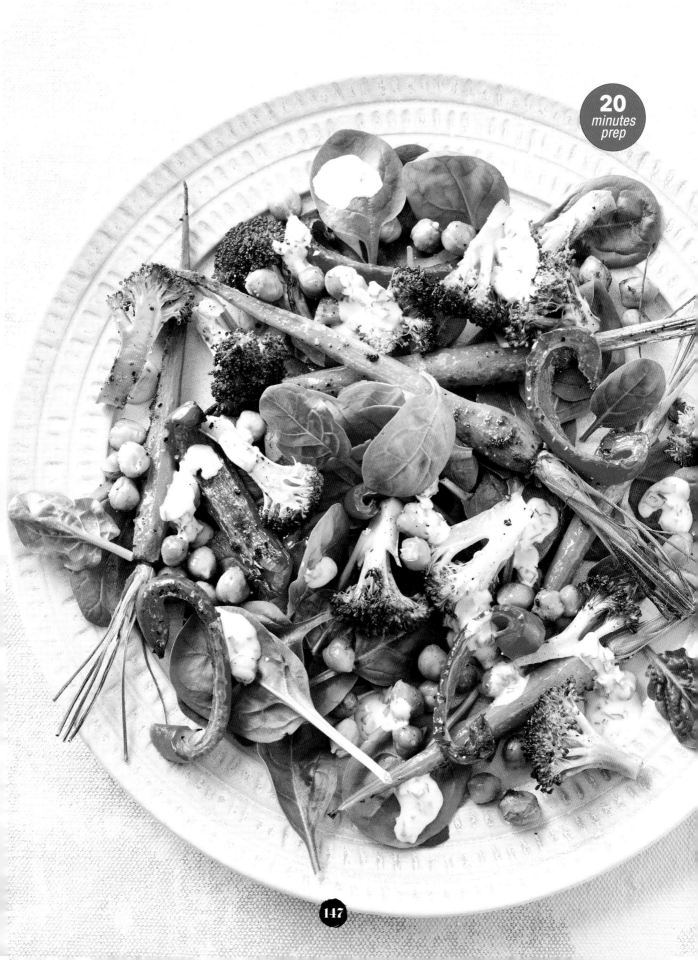

Salmon & Fennel
CITRUS SALAD

Fennel, with its slight aniseed flavour, is the perfect match for rich salmon. Plus, it'll give you fibre and potassium, and is known for aiding digestion.

SERVES 6 **PREP** 20 mins (+ 1 hour marinating & cooling) **COOK** 10 mins

4 oranges
1 lemon, rind finely grated
2 tbs chopped fresh dill
3 (200g each) skinless salmon fillets
250g snow peas, thinly sliced
2 baby fennel bulbs, thinly sliced
120g baby spinach and rocket mix
1 tbs white balsamic vinegar
1 tbs extra virgin olive oil
2 tbs chopped pistachio kernels

1 Finely grate the rind of 1 orange, then juice. Peel and thinly slice the remaining oranges.

2 Combine the lemon rind, orange rind, half the orange juice and 1 tbs dill in a shallow glass or ceramic dish. Add the salmon and turn to coat. Cover and place in fridge for 1 hour to marinate (see note).

3 Preheat a barbecue grill or chargrill pan on medium-high. Drain the marinade from the salmon. Lightly spray the salmon with extra virgin olive oil. Cook the salmon for 2-3 minutes each side for medium or until cooked to your liking. Set aside to cool slightly. Coarsely flake.

4 Place the snow peas in a heatproof bowl. Cover with boiling water. Set aside for 1 minute to blanch. Drain. Refresh under cold running water.

5 Place the snow peas, fennel, spinach and rocket mix and orange slices in a large bowl.

6 Whisk together the vinegar, oil, remaining orange juice and remaining dill in a bowl. Pour half the dressing over the salad and gently toss to combine.

7 Pile the salad onto serving plates and top with the salmon. Drizzle over the remaining dressing and sprinkle with pistachio to serve.

COOK'S NOTE

Don't marinate the salmon for longer than 1 hour, otherwise the juice will start to 'cook' the delicate flesh. Serve with steamed quinoa or freekeh, if you like.

NUTRITION (PER SERVE)

CALS	FAT	SAT FAT	PROTEIN	CARBS
330	18.3g	3.4g	25.7g	13.1g

● EASY ○ QUICK ○ MAKE AHEAD ○ MEAT FREE ● FAMILY FRIENDLY

20+
minutes
prep

★★★★★

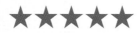
Dill, salmon, snow peas and fennel – four of my favourite things!

FRIDGETUNER

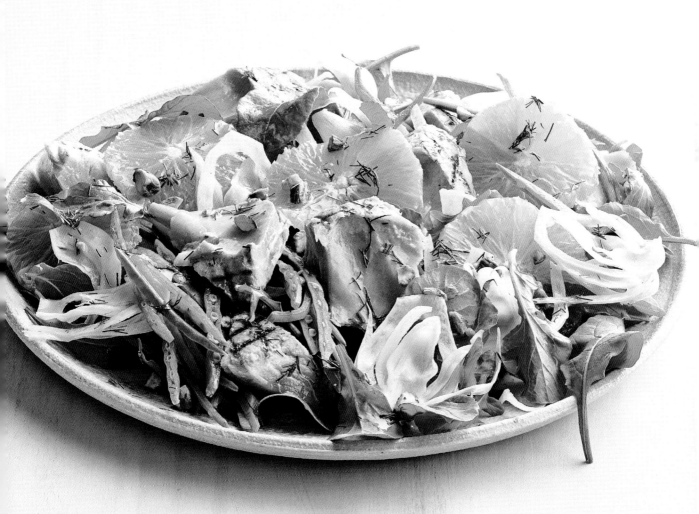

Warm Hazelnut FETA & BARLEY

Barley is a nutritious wholegrain and hazelnuts add healthy fatty acids that promote heart health and anti-inflammatory antioxidants linked to longevity.

SERVES 4 **PREP** 15 mins **COOK** 25 mins

1 large red capsicum, deseeded, cut into 4cm pieces

1 large zucchini, thickly sliced

1 small eggplant, halved lengthways, thickly sliced

220g (1 cup) pearl barley, rinsed, drained

80g baby spinach, coarsely chopped, plus 20g leaves extra

40g (¼ cup) roasted blanched hazelnuts, chopped

50g goat's feta, crumbled

40g (¼ cup) unsweetened dried blueberries (see note)

1½ tbs white balsamic vinegar

1 tbs extra virgin olive oil

1 tsp honey

2 tbs chopped fresh dill

1 Preheat oven to 200°C/180°C fan forced. Line a baking tray with baking paper.

2 Place the capsicum, zucchini and eggplant on prepared tray. Spray with extra virgin olive oil. Roast for 20 minutes or until golden and tender.

3 Meanwhile, cook the barley in a large saucepan of boiling water for 25 minutes or until al dente. Drain.

4 Combine the warm barley, roasted vegetables, spinach, hazelnut, feta and blueberries in a large bowl. Season. Gently toss until combined. Scatter over the extra spinach.

5 Whisk together the vinegar, oil, honey and dill in a bowl then drizzle over the barley mixture. Divide among serving plates.

COOK'S NOTE

Find dried blueberries in the health food aisle at the supermarket.

NUTRITION (PER SERVE)

CALS	FAT	SAT FAT	PROTEIN	CARBS
420	16.6g	3.2g	11.7g	50.6g

★★★★★

I love that fruit and nuts are the star of this dinner show.

FOODSLED

● EASY ○ QUICK ○ MAKE AHEAD ● MEAT-FREE ● FAMILY FRIENDLY

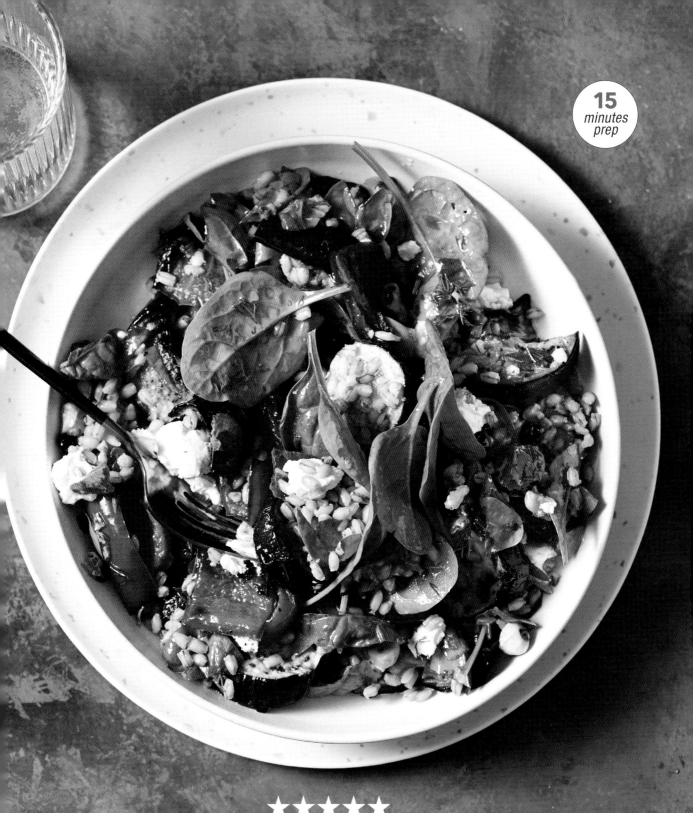

★★★★★

Can never go past goat's cheese! This was a great vego meal.

DRPRETTY

Pickled Grape
GREEN SALAD

Update your classic green leafy salad with pickled grapes. These sweet and salty sensations are also delish on a cheese or charcuterie board.

SERVES 8 (as a side) **PREP** 10 mins (+ 20 mins standing)

1 French shallot, thinly sliced
2 tbs white wine vinegar
2 tbs extra virgin olive oil
2 tsp caster sugar
250g green seedless grapes, stems removed, halved
1 gem lettuce, leaves separated
½ small radicchio lettuce, leaves separated
2 cups watercress sprigs
4 qukes (baby cucumbers), sliced
1 avocado, halved, sliced
½ bunch small red radishes, thinly sliced
60g (⅓ cup) roasted almonds, coarsely chopped

1 Place the shallot in a small bowl. Cover with boiling water. Set aside for 10 minutes (see note). Drain.
2 Combine the vinegar, oil and sugar in a bowl. Add the grapes and shallot. Stir to combine. Set aside for 10 minutes to pickle.
3 Combine the lettuces and watercress in a serving bowl. Top with the quke, avocado and radish. Spoon over the grape mixture. Sprinkle with the almonds. Season and serve.

COOK'S NOTE

Soaking the shallot in boiling water takes away the sharp raw onion taste, leaving it with a more mellow flavour.

NUTRITION (PER SERVE)

CALS	FAT	SAT FAT	PROTEIN	CARBS
150	12g	1.9g	2.5g	7g

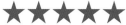

Great salad! The pickled grapes and onions provide an interesting spin on an everyday green salad.
KITEKATO

● EASY ● QUICK ○ MAKE AHEAD ● MEAT FREE ○ FAMILY FRIENDLY

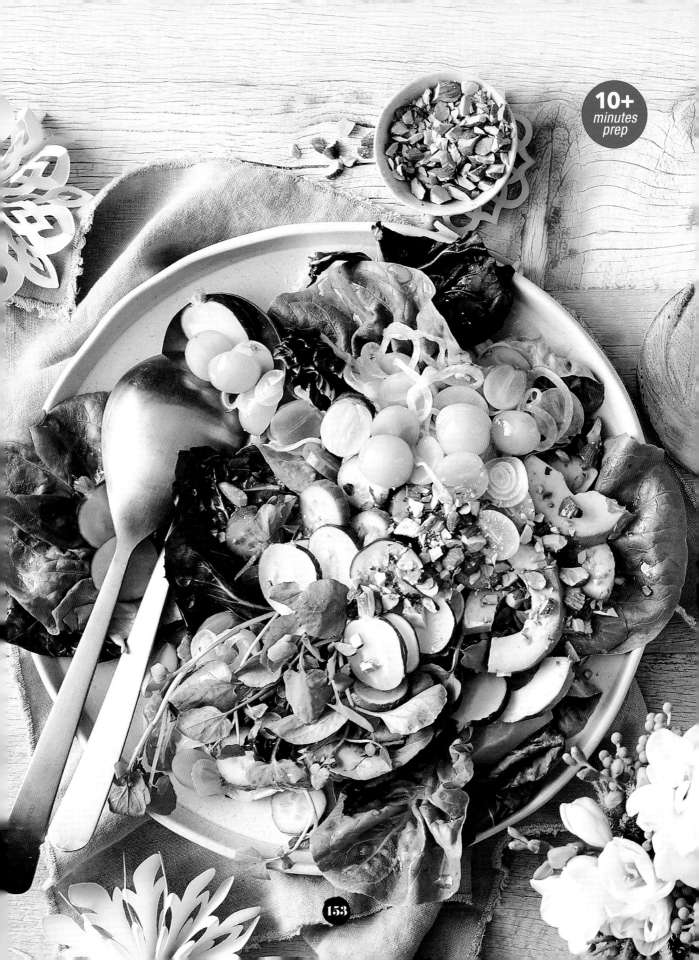

Green Bean & Couscous
CHILLI TUNA

A quick and easy super veg fix is what you need during a busy day.
Fuel up with this winner – the couscous and tuna will keep you going.

SERVES 4 **PREP** 10 mins **COOK** 5 mins

300g green beans, halved
190g (1 cup) wholemeal couscous
250ml (1 cup) boiling water
425g can tuna in chilli oil,
    drained, flaked
200g cherry tomatoes, halved
120g baby spinach and rocket mix
⅔ cup chopped fresh continental
    parsley leaves
60ml (¼ cup) fresh lemon juice
1 tbs extra virgin olive oil

1 Cook the beans in a steamer basket over a saucepan of boiling water for 2-3 minutes or until tender crisp. Drain well.
2 Meanwhile, place the couscous in a large heatproof bowl then pour over the boiling water. Stir to combine. Cover and set aside for 3 minutes or until the liquid is absorbed. Use a fork to separate the grains. Season.
3 Add the beans, tuna, tomato, spinach, rocket and parsley to the couscous. Combine the lemon juice and oil in a jug.
4 Pour the dressing over the couscous mixture and toss to combine. Divide among serving bowls to serve.

COOK'S NOTE

Make ahead without the tuna, spinach and rocket for 4 lunches to take to work. Add a 95g can tuna and 30g spinach and rocket to a single serve on the morning of. Keep chilled until lunchtime.

NUTRITION (PER SERVE)

CALS	FAT	SAT FAT	PROTEIN	CARBS
304	6.4g	1.5g	54.3g	30.7g

★★★★★

Great quick and easy lunch for the work week. Absolutely divine.
SHIRLEEN

● EASY ● QUICK ● MAKE AHEAD ○ MEAT FREE ○ FAMILY FRIENDLY

10 minutes prep

★★★★★
Delicious and tasty.
NICOLEGOODACRE16

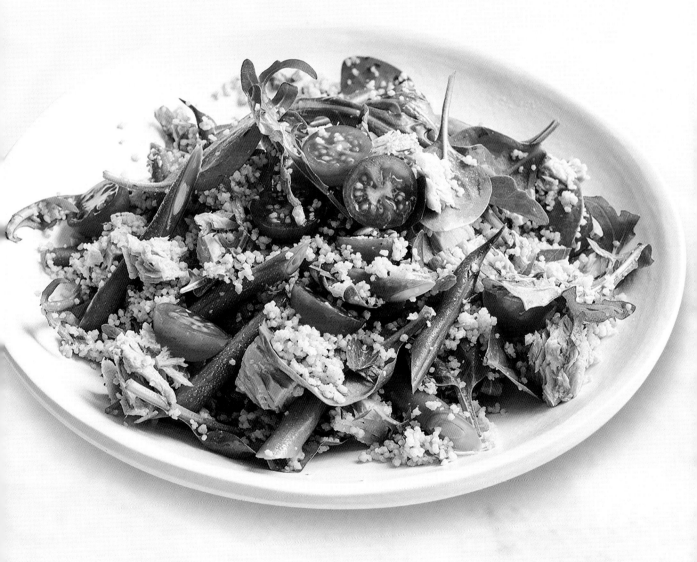

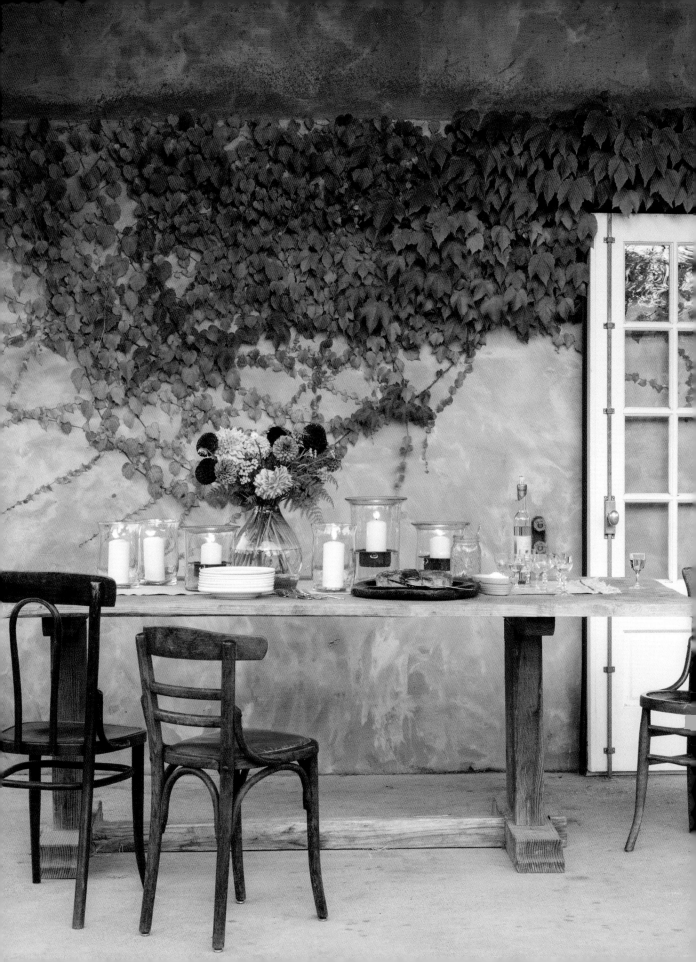

DINNER

MAKE THE MOST OF THE AMAZING PRODUCE AND
PROTEINS AUSTRALIA HAS TO OFFER WITH THIS
BIG AND BEAUTIFUL COLLECTION OF MAINS.

Tomato & Garlic
BRAISED BEANS

Cannellini beans add plant protein to this Mediterranean classic, boosting the overall fibre content of this green bean dream.

SERVES 4 **PREP** 10 mins **COOK** 55 mins

2 tbs extra virgin olive oil
1 brown onion, finely chopped
3 garlic cloves, thinly sliced
1 tsp dried oregano leaves
2 x 400g cans diced tomatoes
400g can cannellini beans, rinsed, drained
450g green beans
90g (⅓ cup) Greek-style yoghurt
1 tsp sumac
4 slices wholegrain sourdough, toasted

1 Heat the oil in a large saucepan over medium heat. Add the onion and cook, stirring, for 5 minutes or until softened. Add the garlic and oregano. Cook, stirring, for 1-2 minutes or until aromatic. Add the tomatoes and stir until combined. Season. Reduce heat to medium-low and simmer for 10 minutes or until the mixture thickens slightly. Add the cannellini beans and simmer for 5 minutes or until heated through.
2 Arrange the green beans in a single layer on top of the tomato mixture. Cover and simmer for 30 minutes or until the beans are tender.
3 Meanwhile, combine the yoghurt and sumac in a small bowl.
4 Dollop the sumac yoghurt over the braised beans and serve with the toast.

COOK'S NOTE

This is a complete meal (with the toast), but you could serve it with wholemeal couscous instead, if you prefer.

NUTRITION (PER SERVE)

CALS	FAT	SAT FAT	PROTEIN	CARBS
340	12g	2.4g	14.3g	35.5g

★★★★★

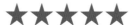
I was amazed how full I felt after eating this. Between the cannellini beans and the toast, it was super satisfying.

FANCY FOODIE

● EASY ○ QUICK ○ MAKE AHEAD ● MEAT FREE ● FAMILY FRIENDLY

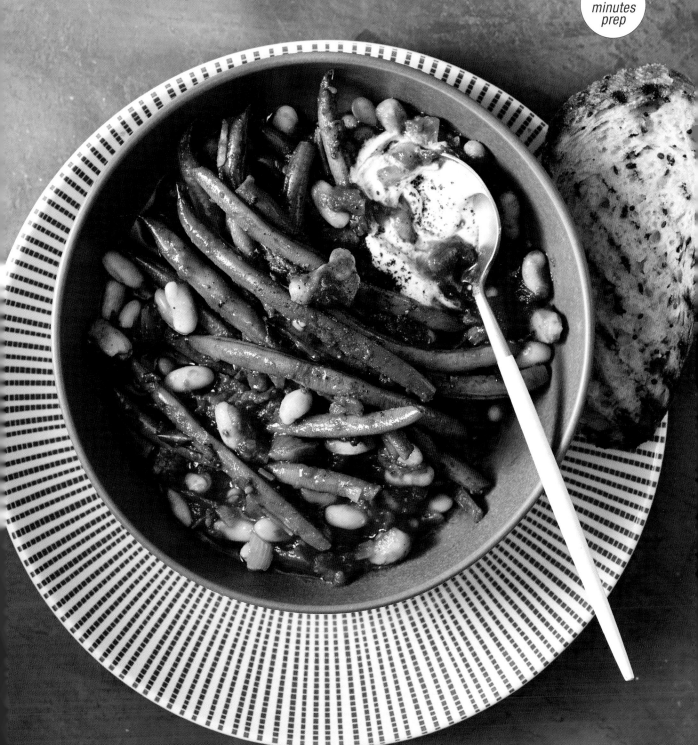

Acqua Pazza
BARRAMUNDI

Simple flavours shine in this Italian fish dish that's reached super veg status! Added bonus: it's full of heart-healthy ingredients.

SERVES 4 **PREP** 20 mins **COOK** 25 mins

1 tbs extra virgin olive oil, plus extra to serve

1 leek, thinly sliced

1 fennel bulb, thinly sliced

3 garlic cloves, thinly sliced

1 long fresh red chilli, deseeded, thinly sliced

125ml (½ cup) dry white wine

320g mixed cherry tomatoes, halved

55g (⅓ cup) pitted kalamata olives

4 (about 125g each) barramundi fillets, skin on

125ml (½ cup) salt-reduced chicken or fish stock

2 tbs chopped fresh continental parsley leaves

4 slices wholegrain sourdough bread, toasted

1 Heat the oil in a large frying pan over medium heat. Add the leek and fennel. Cook, stirring, for 5 minutes or until softened. Add the garlic and chilli. Cook, stirring, for 1 minute or until aromatic.

2 Pour in the wine. Bring to a simmer. Cook for 1-2 minutes. Add the tomato and olives. Simmer for 2 minutes then add the barramundi, stock and 200ml water. Bring to the boil. Reduce heat to low. Simmer, covered, for 8-10 minutes or until the fish is cooked through. Season. Sprinkle with the parsley. Drizzle over extra oil and serve with the toast.

COOK'S NOTE

Try serving this on a bed of cooked quinoa or wholemeal couscous and omit the bread.

NUTRITION (PER SERVE)

CALS	FAT	SAT FAT	PROTEIN	CARBS
351	9.8g	1.6g	32g	23.2g

★★★★★

Another favourite. The flavours are sensational and linger long after you have finished eating it. We served ours with couscous. Absolutely will be repeating. Thank you. **MICHELLE**

● **EASY** ○ QUICK ○ MAKE AHEAD ○ MEAT FREE ○ FAMILY FRIENDLY

★★★★★

Delicious recipe. Really easy. Fish tasted beautiful steamed with the yummy sauce. Served with couscous.

MAG.GANDER

20 minutes prep

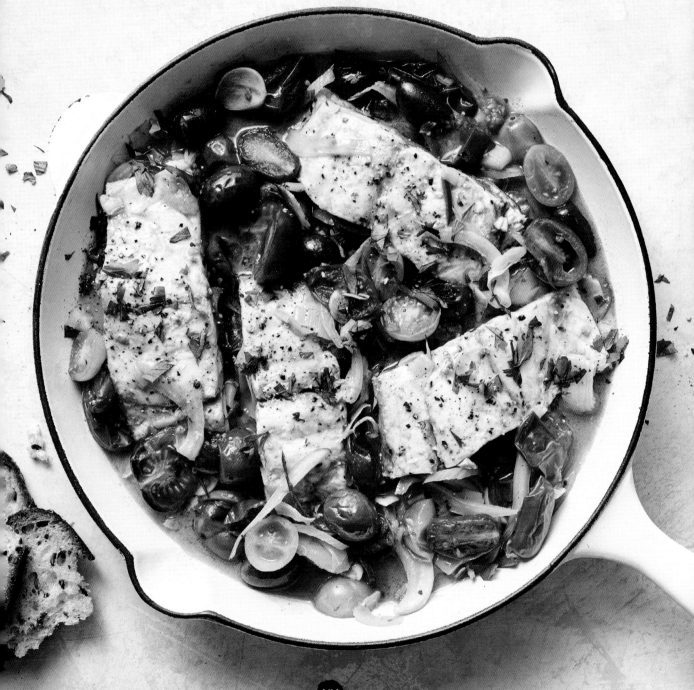

Silverbeet Pesto
ORECCHIETTE

Try silverbeet as a twist on regular basil pesto. This speedy pasta is your saviour for a midweek meal for the hungry hordes.

SERVES 4 **PREP** 10 mins **COOK** 15 mins

1 small bunch silverbeet, stems removed
400g dried orecchiette pasta
50g pine nuts, toasted
1 large garlic clove, chopped
1 tsp finely grated lemon rind
120g Greek feta, crumbled
60ml (¼ cup) extra virgin olive oil, plus extra to drizzle
1½ tbs fresh lemon juice

1 Bring a large saucepan of water to the boil over high heat. Season with salt. Add the silverbeet leaves. Cook for 1 minute 30 seconds or until just blanched. Use a slotted spoon to transfer the silverbeet to a colander. Refresh under cold running water. Dry well.

2 Cook the pasta in a large saucepan of salted boiling water until al dente. Drain, reserving 80ml (⅓ cupful) cooking liquid. Return the pasta and reserved liquid to the pan.

3 Meanwhile, reserve 1 tbs pine nuts. Place the silverbeet, garlic, lemon rind and remaining pine nuts in a food processor. Process until finely chopped. Add half of the feta. Process until smooth. Whisk together the oil, lemon juice and 1 tbs water in a jug. With the processor motor running, add the oil mixture to the silverbeet mixture in a thin, steady stream until smooth. Season.

4 Add the silverbeet pesto to the pasta mixture and gently toss until combined. Sprinkle with the reserved pine nuts and remaining feta. Drizzle over some extra oil.

COOK'S NOTE

Dried orecchiette to spare? Cook a small batch and dress with a vinaigrette. Toss through canned tuna and fresh herbs as an easy lunch for one.

NUTRITION (PER SERVE)

CALS	FAT	SAT FAT	PROTEIN	CARBS
696	36g	8g	19g	72g

★ ★ ★ ★ ★

Very tasty crowd pleaser. Easy too. **COLECORP43**

● EASY   ● QUICK   ○ MAKE AHEAD   ● MEAT FREE   ● FAMILY FRIENDLY

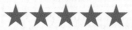

★ ★ ★ ★ ★

Quick & easy with minimal cooking! Great recipe.

TDAVEY86

10 minutes prep

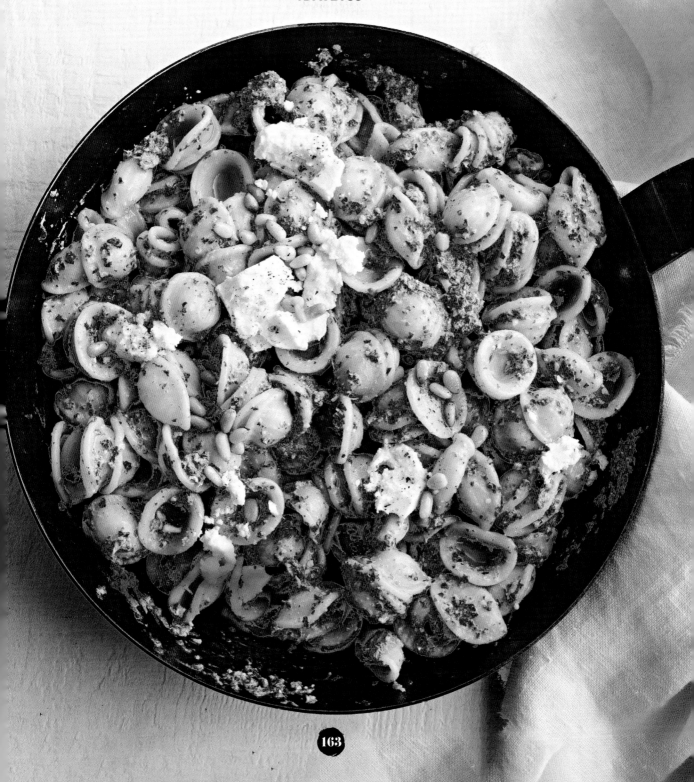

Lentil Tabouli with
DUKKAH PORK

Sealing pork cutlets in a warming dukkah spice keeps them moist and tender. Plus, it's a simple way to add big flavour in a flash.

SERVES 4 **PREP** 5 mins (+ 5 mins resting) **COOK** 10 mins

4 (about 125g each) pork loin cutlets, excess fat trimmed

1 tbs dukkah

3 ripe tomatoes

1 Lebanese cucumber

1 bunch fresh continental parsley, leaves picked

1 bunch fresh mint, leaves picked

3 green shallots

400g can brown lentils, rinsed, drained

2 tbs fresh lemon juice

2 tbs extra virgin olive oil, plus extra to drizzle

90g (⅓ cup) Greek-style yoghurt

1 small garlic clove, crushed

1 Preheat a barbecue grill or chargrill pan on medium. Sprinkle the pork all over with the dukkah. Spray with extra virgin olive oil. Cook for 5 minutes each side or until golden. Set aside for 5 minutes to rest.

2 Meanwhile, finely chop the tomatoes, cucumber, parsley and mint. Slice the shallots. Combine in a large bowl with the lentils, lemon juice and oil. Season and stir to combine. Combine the yoghurt and garlic in a small bowl.

3 Divide the tabouli and pork among serving plates. Drizzle over a little extra oil and season with pepper. Serve with the garlic yoghurt.

NUTRITION (PER SERVE)

CALS	FAT	SAT FAT	PROTEIN	CARBS
407	20.4g	5.1g	35.7g	15.7g

COOK'S NOTE

Get ahead by picking the herbs from the stems up to a day ahead. Keep in a bowl of water in the fridge, then drain and whiz in a salad spinner to dry thoroughly. Serve with wholemeal pita bread, if you like.

★★★★★

So fresh! Inspired to try crumbing other proteins in dukkah.
WAFFLEISO

● EASY ● QUICK ○ MAKE AHEAD ○ MEAT FREE ● FAMILY FRIENDLY

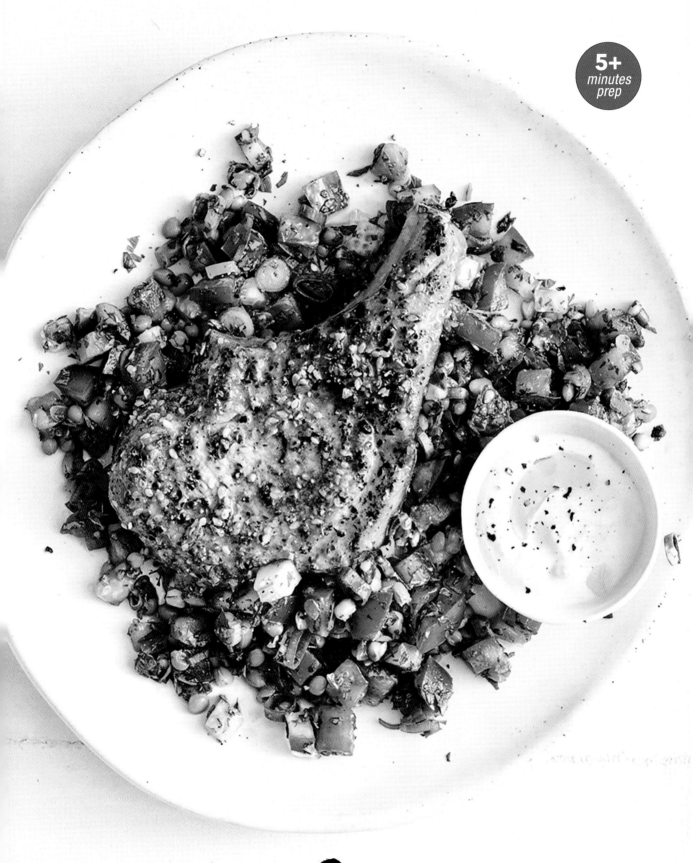

Super Green
QUINOA PILAF

This grain dish is brimming with superfoods. Wholegrain quinoa, broccolini and corn are rich sources of plant protein, and that's just the start!

SERVES 4 **PREP** 20 mins **COOK** 20 mins

1 tbs extra virgin olive oil
1 brown onion, finely chopped
2 garlic cloves, crushed
200g (1 cup) quinoa, rinsed, drained
500ml (2 cups) salt-reduced
   vegetable stock
1 bunch broccolini, trimmed, cut into
   3cm pieces, stems halved if large
1 large corncob, kernels removed
1 bunch asparagus, trimmed,
   sliced lengthways
150g sugar snap peas,
   halved lengthways
100g baby spinach
2 tbs chopped pistachio kernels
2 tbs pomegranate arils
Lime wedges, to serve

1 Heat the oil in a large saucepan over high heat. Add the onion and cook, stirring occasionally, for 5 minutes or until softened. Add the garlic and cook, stirring, for 1 minute or until aromatic.
2 Add the quinoa and stock. Bring to boil then reduce heat to low. Cover and simmer for 12 minutes or until almost all the stock is absorbed. Add the broccolini, corn, asparagus and sugar snap peas. Stir to combine. Cover and cook for 2 minutes or until all the stock is absorbed. Remove from heat. Set aside, covered, for 3-4 minutes to steam.
3 Stir through the spinach and season. Divide the pilaf among serving plates. Sprinkle with the pistachios and pomegranate. Serve with lime wedges to squeeze over.

COOK'S NOTE

Make a double batch of this pilaf for an easy, nourishing lunch the next day.

NUTRITION (PER SERVE)

CALS	FAT	SAT FAT	PROTEIN	CARBS
484	21.8g	9.7g	22g	46.4g

★★★★★

I thought the best bit was that everything basically gets thrown in the saucepan to cook. That was until I tucked in – yum! **VIOLAPARMESAN**

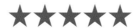

● EASY ○ QUICK ● MAKE AHEAD ● MEAT FREE ● FAMILY FRIENDLY

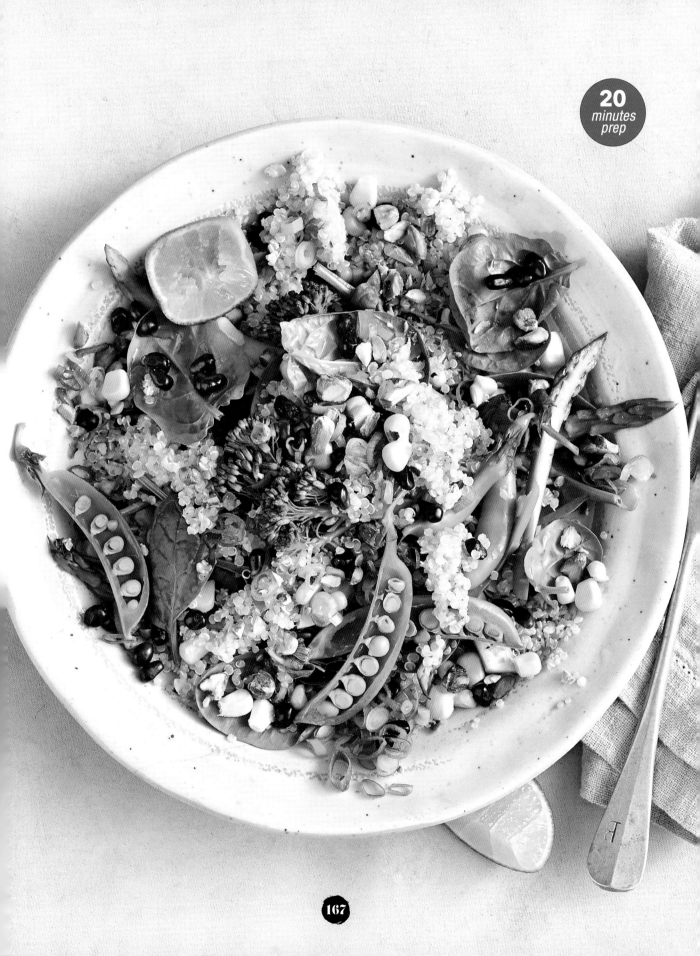

Tomato & Potato
SNAPPER BAKE

Oh snap! This tray bake is big on all things Mediterranean. Plus, bringing a whole fish to the table is going to impress, we guarantee it.

SERVES 8 **PREP** 25 mins **COOK** 1 hour

400g cocktail truss tomatoes
160ml (⅔ cup) dry white wine
2 tbs fresh lemon juice (see note)
4 garlic cloves, crushed
2 tsp ground coriander
1 tsp sweet paprika
160ml (⅔ cup) extra virgin olive oil
1kg red-skinned potatoes, unpeeled,
   cut into 1cm slices
⅔ cup fresh oregano leaves,
   plus extra to serve
⅔ cup fresh dill, plus extra to serve
2 tsp finely grated lemon rind
1 tsp caraway seeds
1.5kg whole cleaned snapper
65g (⅓ cup) kalamata olives
2 tbs drained capers, rinsed
Lemon wedges, to serve

1 Preheat oven to 200°C/180°C fan forced. Grease a large baking tray with a rim.
2 Pull half of the tomatoes off the vine. Place in a large bowl. Use your hands to crush the tomatoes. Add the wine, lemon juice, garlic, coriander, paprika and 1 tbs oil. Season and stir to combine. Add the potato and toss to combine. Transfer the potato mixture to prepared tray. Roast for 30 minutes.
3 Meanwhile, place the oregano, dill, lemon rind, caraway seeds and remaining oil in a small food processor. Season. Process until finely chopped. Cut 4 slits on each side of the snapper. Rub the dill mixture into the cavity and slits.
4 Place the fish on top of the potato mixture and roast for 15 minutes.
5 Add the olives, capers and remaining tomatoes still on the vine to the tray. Roast for a further 15 minutes or until the snapper is cooked through. Sprinkle with extra oregano and dill. Serve with lemon wedges to squeeze over.

COOK'S NOTE

Grate the lemon rind before you cut the lemon in half to squeeze the juice – much easier! Watch out for fish bones as you eat. Use your fork to gently slide the flesh off the spine and bones.

NUTRITION (PER SERVE)

CALS	FAT	SAT FAT	PROTEIN	CARBS
359	11.5g	2.1g	42.3g	16.1g

● EASY ○ QUICK ○ MAKE AHEAD ○ MEAT FREE ○ FAMILY FRIENDLY

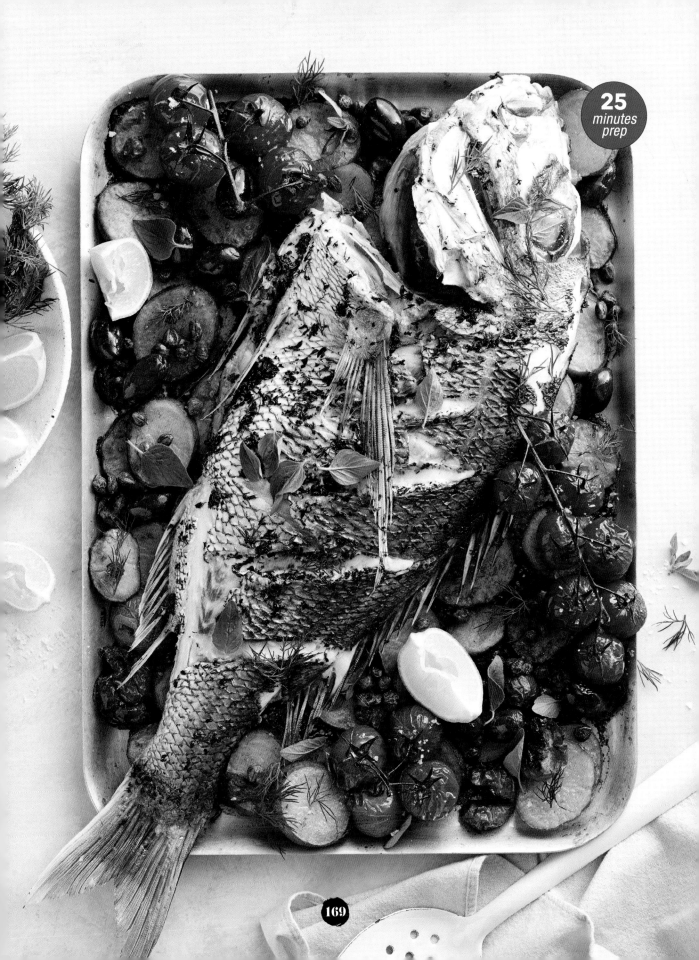

25
minutes
prep

169

Spiced Chickpea
PORK STEW

This oven-baked casserole is just what the doctor ordered. A hearty helping served with couscous and steamed veg will help boost your immunity.

SERVES 4 **PREP** 15 mins **COOK** 1 hour 50 mins

2 tsp extra virgin olive oil

500g trimmed lean pork shoulder, chopped

1 large red onion, thinly sliced

2 celery sticks, finely chopped

3 carrots, peeled, sliced

2 garlic cloves, thinly sliced

2 tsp finely grated fresh ginger

1 tsp ground cumin

½ tsp ground cinnamon

½ tsp ground turmeric

250ml (1 cup) salt-reduced chicken stock

400g can diced tomatoes

400g can chickpeas, rinsed, drained

2 tbs raisins

Micro herbs, steamed wholemeal couscous and steamed greens, to serve

1 Preheat oven to 180°C/160°C fan forced.

2 Heat half the oil in a large deep frying pan over high heat. In 2 batches, cook the pork, stirring, for 3-4 minutes or until browned. Transfer to a large ovenproof casserole dish.

3 Heat the remaining oil in the pan over medium heat. Add the onion, celery and carrot. Cook, stirring, for 5 minutes or until softened. Add the garlic, ginger, cumin, cinnamon and turmeric. Cook, stirring, for 1 minute. Add the stock, tomatoes, chickpeas and raisins. Bring to the boil.

4 Pour the tomato mixture over the pork. Cover and roast for 1 hour 30 minutes or until the pork is very tender. Season. Divide the stew among serving bowls. Sprinkle with micro herbs, season and serve with couscous and steamed greens.

COOK'S NOTE

This stew can be made ahead. Cover and place in the fridge for up to 3 days or freeze in airtight containers for up to 1 month.

NUTRITION (PER SERVE)

CALS	FAT	SAT FAT	PROTEIN	CARBS
392	6g	1g	38g	40g

★★★★★

I was drawn in by all the health benefits of this stew. Yum! A filling, easy one for when it's chilly. **HARMONYPUFFIN**

● EASY　○ QUICK　● MAKE AHEAD　○ MEAT FREE　● FAMILY FRIENDLY

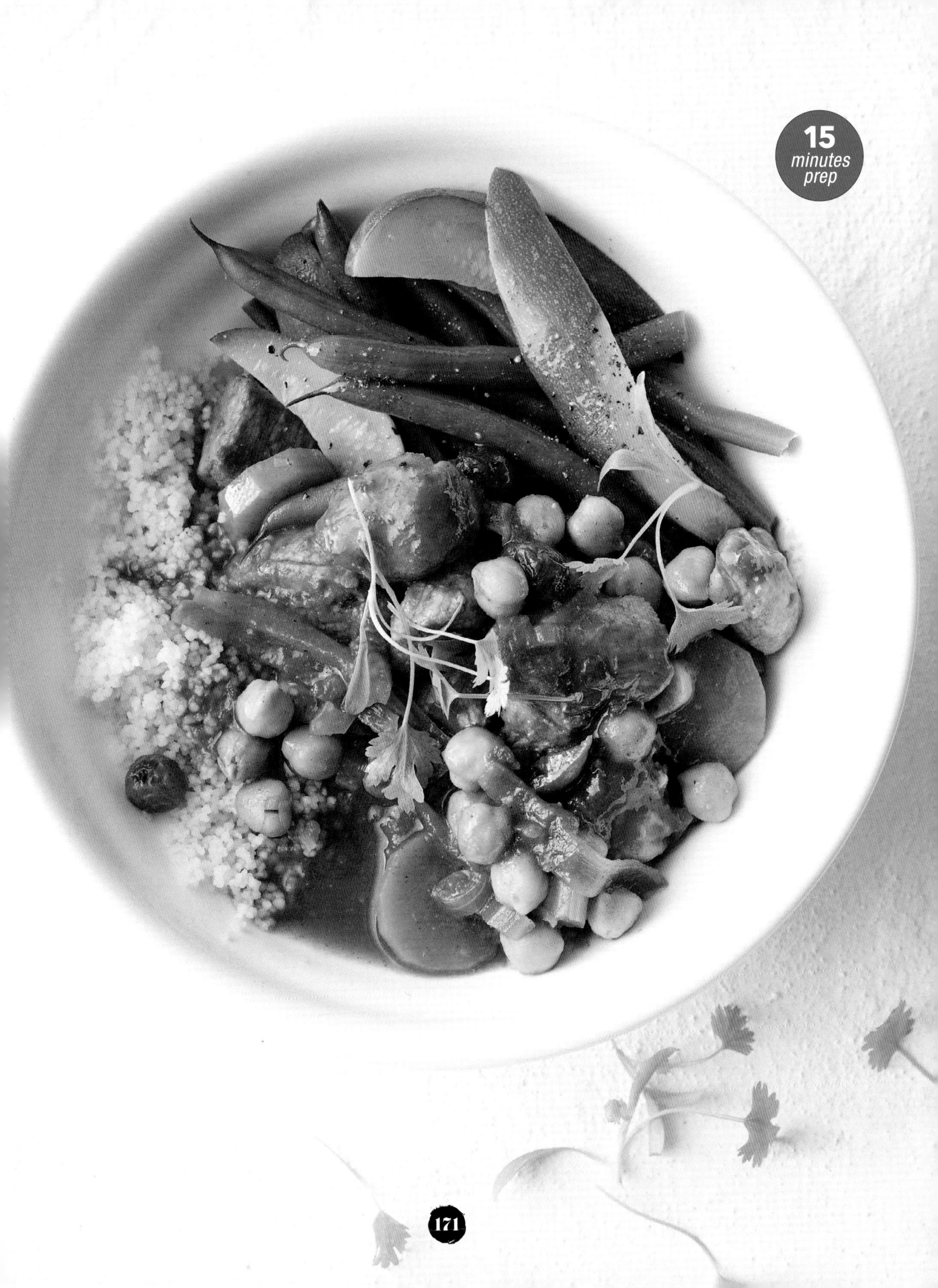
15
minutes
prep

Buckwheat & Roast
CAULI PASTA

Wholegrain pasta gives you more nutritional bang for your buck. Buckwheat pasta is rich in antioxidants that help lower cholesterol and blood pressure.

SERVES 4 **PREP** 15 mins **COOK** 25 mins

1 small head (about 700g) cauliflower, cut into florets
2 tbs currants
2 tsp balsamic vinegar
200g dried buckwheat penne pasta
1 tbs extra virgin olive oil
4 green shallots, thinly sliced
2 garlic cloves, crushed
2 tsp finely grated lemon rind
400g can chickpeas, rinsed, drained
80ml (⅓ cup) salt-reduced vegetable stock
100g baby spinach
¼ cup chopped fresh continental parsley, plus extra leaves to serve
1 tbs fresh lemon juice

1 Preheat oven to 200°C/180°C fan forced. Line a baking tray with baking paper.
2 Place the cauliflower on prepared tray and spray lightly with extra virgin olive oil. Roast for 20-25 minutes or until golden. Place the currants and vinegar in a small bowl. Set aside to soak.
3 Meanwhile, cook the pasta in a large saucepan of lightly salted boiling water following packet directions or until al dente. Drain and return to the pan.
4 Heat 2 tsp oil in a large non-stick frying pan over medium heat. Add the shallot, garlic and lemon rind. Cook, stirring, for 1 minute. Add the currant mixture and cook for 1 minute. Add the chickpeas and stock. Simmer for 2 minutes or until reduced by half. Stir in the spinach until wilted.
5 Add the chickpea mixture, roast cauliflower, parsley, lemon juice and remaining 2 tsp oil to the pasta. Toss until well combined. Season. Divide among serving plates and serve sprinkled with extra parsley.

COOK'S NOTE

Roast the cauliflower up to 1 day ahead. Keep in the fridge, but reheat in the microwave before using.

NUTRITION (PER SERVE)

CALS	FAT	SAT FAT	PROTEIN	CARBS
363	7g	1g	13g	54g

★★★★★

Superb recipe. The nutty flavour of the baked cauliflower beautifully offsets the acid sweetness of the currant-balsamic mixture. **SHIRLEEN**

● EASY   ○ QUICK   ○ MAKE AHEAD   ● MEAT FREE   ● FAMILY FRIENDLY

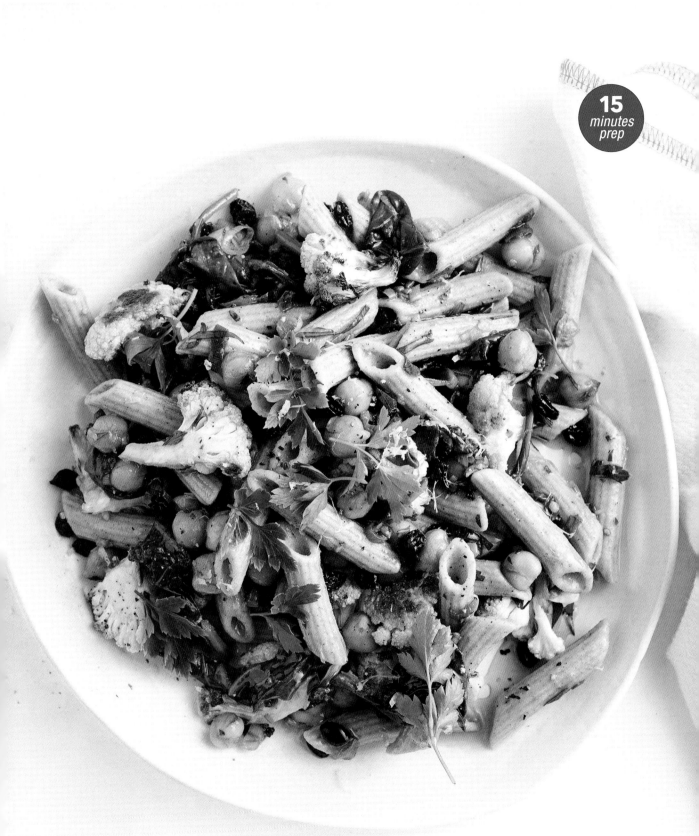

Salmon with
BEAN AGRODOLCE

By letting vegies and legumes play a bigger role on the dinner plate, you can easily make the changes to adopt a way of eating that's better for you.

SERVES 4 **PREP** 10 mins **COOK** 20 mins

2½ tbs extra virgin olive oil

1 red onion, finely chopped

1 garlic clove, crushed

2½ tbs currants

2 large zucchini, halved lengthways, sliced diagonally, cut into batons

300g tomato medley mix, halved

400g can cannellini beans, rinsed, drained

2 tbs red wine vinegar

1 tsp caster sugar

⅓ cup fresh continental parsley leaves

4 (about 120g each) salmon fillets, skin on

1 Heat 2 tbs oil in a large frying pan over medium heat. Add the onion and cook, stirring, for 3 minutes or until softened. Add the garlic and currants. Cook, stirring, for 1 minute.

2 Increase heat to medium-high. Add the zucchini and cook, stirring, for 5 minutes or until just tender. Add the tomato and cook, stirring, for 1 minute. Add the beans and cook, stirring, for 2 minutes or until heated through.

3 Pour in the vinegar and sugar. Simmer for 30 seconds then remove from heat. Season well. Stir through the parsley and cover to keep warm.

4 Heat the remaining oil in a large non-stick frying pan over medium heat. Pat dry the salmon. Season the skin well with salt. Cook, skin-side down, for 3-4 minutes or until crisp. Turn. Cook for a further 2 minutes for medium or until cooked to your liking.

5 Transfer the bean mixture to a serving platter. Arrange the salmon on top to serve.

COOK'S NOTE

Use up any leftover currants by sauteeing with silverbeet and a splash of vinegar. Mix with fresh ricotta and cinnamon for a savoury crepe filling.

NUTRITION (PER SERVE)

CALS	FAT	SAT FAT	PROTEIN	CARBS
476	28.4g	5.2g	31.9g	18.5g

● EASY ● QUICK ○ MAKE AHEAD ○ MEAT FREE ● FAMILY FRIENDLY

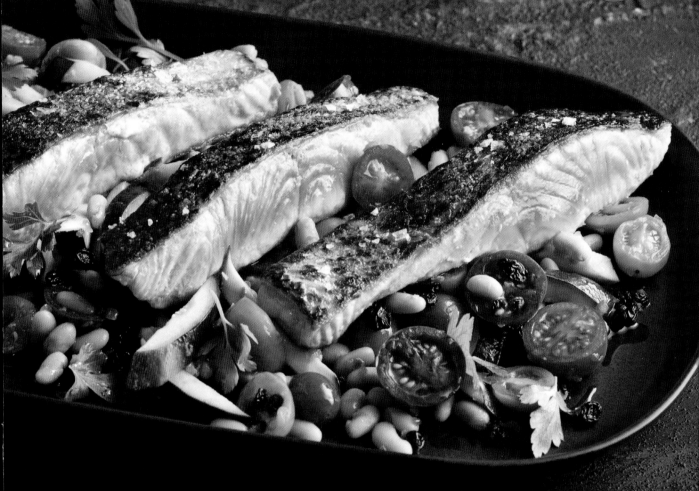

10
minutes
prep

★★★★★
Added various other vegies too. Delicious.
CYNDI84

Cauliflower & Olive
LAMB PILAF

While your red meat intake needs to be limited to less than two serves a week, make one of those meals a vegie-full affair for maximum nourishment!

SERVES 4 **PREP** 10 mins (+ 10 mins marinating) **COOK** 10 mins

2 (about 500g) lamb backstraps

2 tbs extra virgin olive oil

2 tsp ground cumin

2 tsp ground coriander

1 small (about 700g) head cauliflower, cut into florets

120g chilli and garlic marinated green olives, halved

2 tbs currants

1 large lemon, rind finely grated, juiced

1 tsp honey

3 green shallots, thinly sliced

1 cup firmly packed mixed fresh herb leaves (such as parsley, coriander and mint)

Greek-style yoghurt, to serve (optional)

Toasted pine nuts, to serve

1 Place the lamb on a plate. Add 2 tsp oil, 1 tsp cumin and 1 tsp ground coriander. Season then turn to coat. Set aside for 10 minutes to marinate.

2 Meanwhile, place the cauliflower in a food processor and process until finely chopped. Heat the remaining oil in a large frying pan over medium-high heat. Add the olives and currants. Cook, stirring, for 1 minute. Add the lemon rind and remaining cumin and ground coriander. Cook, stirring, for 1 minute. Add the cauliflower. Cook, stirring, for 2 minutes. Season well. Pour in half the lemon juice. Cover and cook, stirring occasionally, for 3-4 minutes or until just tender. Set aside to cool slightly.

3 Heat a non-stick frying pan over medium heat. Cook the lamb, turning, for 6 minutes for medium or until cooked to your liking. Remove pan from heat. Drizzle over the honey and remaining lemon juice. Set aside for 3 minutes to rest then slice the lamb.

4 Stir the shallot and herbs into the cauliflower mixture. Divide among serving plates. Top with the lamb and yoghurt, if using. Drizzle over pan juices and sprinkle with pine nuts.

COOK'S NOTE

Marinated olives are a quick and easy way to add loads of flavour. Toss through salads (along with some of the oil from the tub) or put on pizza.

NUTRITION (PER SERVE)

CALS	FAT	SAT FAT	PROTEIN	CARBS
387	22.6g	4.6g	30.1g	13.5g

● EASY ● QUICK ○ MAKE AHEAD ○ MEAT FREE ○ FAMILY FRIENDLY

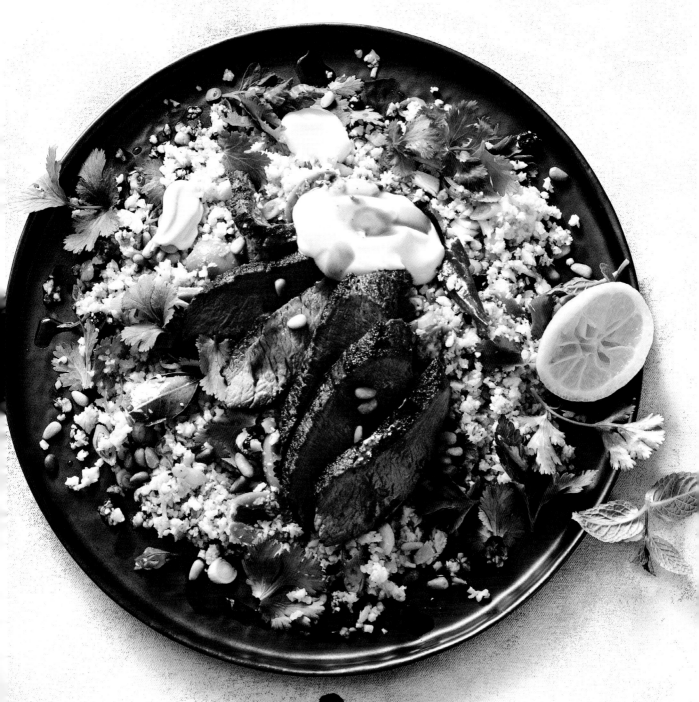

10+
minutes prep

★ ★ ★ ★ ★
Made this tonight as it was the dish of the day.
All I can say is yum! **TANYASCOTT**

Beetroot & Thyme
SPANAKOPITA

This twist on the Greek filo bake goes bold with fresh beetroot. The sprinkling of nutmeg brings out its sweetness. And gotta love that crispy pastry!

SERVES 6 **PREP** 25 mins (+ cooling) **COOK** 55 mins

1½ tbs extra virgin olive oil
½ red onion, finely chopped
3 garlic cloves, crushed
1½ tbs fresh thyme leaves
1 bunch beetroot, peeled, cut into 1cm pieces, leaves washed and thinly sliced
3 tsp honey
3 tsp red wine vinegar
500g fresh ricotta, crumbled
200g Greek feta, crumbled
4 eggs
¼ tsp freshly grated or ground nutmeg
10 sheets filo pastry
3 tsp mixed seeds

1 Preheat oven to 200°C/180°C fan forced. Grease a 18 x 24cm baking dish with oil.
2 Heat the oil in a large non-stick frying pan over medium heat. Add the onion, garlic and 1 tbs thyme. Cook, stirring, for 2 minutes or until softened.
3 Add the beetroot. Cover and cook, stirring occasionally, for 12 minutes or until tender crisp. Add the honey and vinegar. Season well. Cook, stirring, for 3-4 minutes or until the liquid evaporates. Stir in the beetroot leaves. Cook until wilted. Transfer to a colander to drain and cool completely.
4 Combine the ricotta, feta, eggs and nutmeg in a large bowl. Season. Stir in the beetroot mixture until just combined.
5 Place the filo on a clean work surface. Cover with a dry tea towel then a damp tea towel (this will prevent it from drying out). Lightly spray 1 filo sheet with extra virgin olive oil. Top with another sheet and spray with oil. Repeat with 1 more sheet. Lay the filo stack in prepared dish, allowing filo to overhang the edges. Repeat with another 3 filo sheets, laying in the dish at right angles to the first stack. Spoon over the beetroot mixture.
6 Lay the remaining filo sheets over the beetroot mixture, spraying with oil between the sheets. Trim a 1cm border around the edges. Tuck in the overhanging edges. Score diagonally. Sprinkle with the seeds and remaining thyme. Lightly spray with oil. Bake for 30-35 minutes or until crisp.

COOK'S NOTE

Beetroot leaves need not go to waste – they're delicious and nutritious! Try them sauteed in extra virgin olive oil and garlic as a tasty side.

NUTRITION (PER SERVE)

CALS	FAT	SAT FAT	PROTEIN	CARBS
461	29g	12g	23g	25g

○ EASY ○ QUICK ○ MAKE AHEAD ● MEAT FREE ● FAMILY FRIENDLY

★★★★★

Not difficult to cook and super flavoursome!
Definitely an easy favourite.

JACKPEDERSEN97

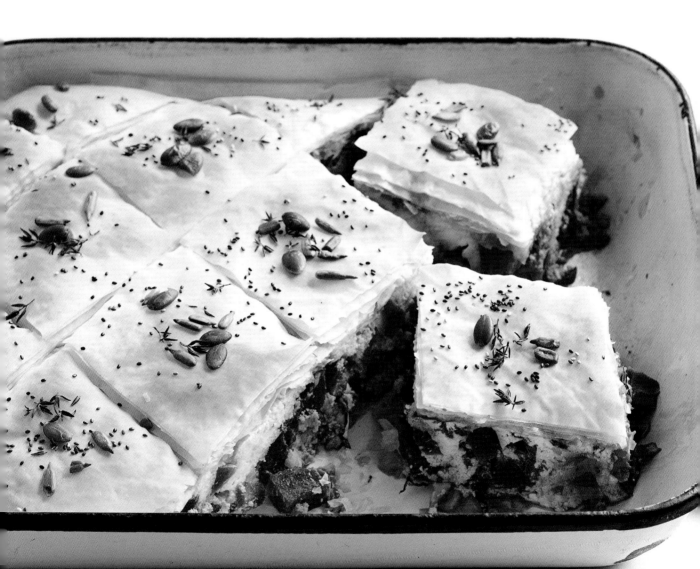

Crispy Caper
LEMON SNAPPER

Broad beans and peas – your friends in the freezer – are what you should reach for on busy weeknights for a crunchy hit of nutrients!

SERVES 4 **PREP** 30 mins **COOK** 10 mins

360g (2 cups) frozen broad beans
150g (1 cup) frozen baby peas
400g can lentils, rinsed, drained
1 small zucchini, very thinly sliced
½ small red onion, thinly sliced
¼ cup fresh dill
2½ tbs extra virgin olive oil
4 (150g each) snapper fillets, skin on
2 tbs baby capers, rinsed, drained
1 tbs finely chopped fresh chives
2 tsp finely grated lemon rind
60ml (¼ cup) fresh lemon juice
Lemon wedges, to serve

1 Cook the broad beans and peas in a large saucepan of boiling water for 3 minutes or until bright green and tender. Drain. Refresh under cold running water. Peel the beans. Transfer to a bowl along with the peas. Add the lentils, zucchini, onion and dill. Toss to combine.

2 Meanwhile, heat 2 tsp oil in a frying pan over medium-high heat. Cook the fish, skin-side down, for 3 minutes. Turn and cook a further 3 minutes or until browned and just cooked through. Transfer to a plate and cover loosely with foil to keep warm.

3 Add the capers and remaining oil to the pan. Cook over medium-high heat, stirring occasionally, for 1 minute or until golden and crisp. Remove from heat. Stir in the chives, lemon rind and juice.

4 Divide the lentil mixture among serving plates. Top with the fish. Spoon over the dressing and season. Serve with lemon wedges to squeeze over.

COOK'S NOTE

Use any type of fish fillet you like in this dish. Find out what is in season and local – it will be cheaper and at its best nutritionally. Serve with steamed freekeh or barley, if you like.

NUTRITION (PER SERVE)

CALS	FAT	SAT FAT	PROTEIN	CARBS
412	15g	2.5g	43.1g	18.1g

★★★★★

Fresh and delicious. Very easy to make. Looks great as well.
CHEZWHITTA

○ EASY   ○ QUICK   ○ MAKE AHEAD   ○ MEAT FREE   ● FAMILY FRIENDLY

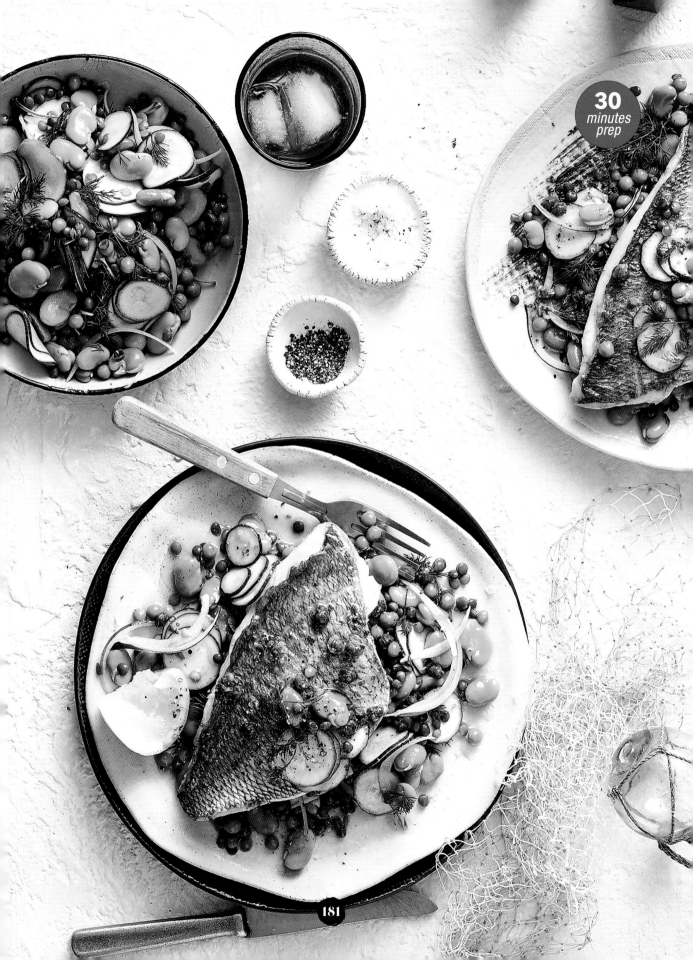

30
*minutes
prep*

181

Pumpkin & Herb
SPICED BEEF

Make dinner nutritious and satisfying by packing it with veg, protein and fibre. Rump steak is a lean cut and so the healthier choice.

SERVES 4 **PREP** 20 mins **COOK** 30 mins

500g peeled and deseeded pumpkin, cut into 2cm pieces
½ tsp ground cumin
½ tsp ground paprika
¼ tsp ground cinnamon
400g beef rump steak, excess fat trimmed
250g green beans, sliced
400g can chickpeas, rinsed, drained
½ cup fresh mint leaves
½ cup fresh continental parsley leaves
2 tbs flaked almonds, lightly toasted (see note)
2 tsp tahini
1 tbs fresh lemon juice
1 tbs hot water
1 tsp honey

1 Preheat oven to 200°C/180°C fan forced. Line a baking tray with baking paper.

2 Place the pumpkin on prepared tray and spray with extra virgin olive oil. Roast for 25 minutes or until tender.

3 Meanwhile, preheat a barbecue grill or chargrill pan on high. Combine the cumin, paprika and cinnamon in a bowl. Sprinkle the spice mixture on both sides of the steak and rub to coat. Lightly spray with oil. Cook the steaks for 2-3 minutes each side for medium or until cooked to your liking. Transfer to a plate. Cover loosely with foil and set aside for 3 minutes to rest. Thinly slice the steak.

4 Place the beans in a steamer over a saucepan of simmering water. Cover and steam for 2 minutes or until tender crisp. Drain. Refresh under cold running water.

5 Place the beans, pumpkin, chickpeas, mint, parsley and almonds in a large bowl. Season.

6 Whisk together the tahini, lemon juice, hot water and honey in a small bowl. Add the dressing to the salad and gently toss to combine. Divide among serving bowls. Top with the steak to serve.

COOK'S NOTE

To toast the almonds, stir them in a dry frying pan over medium heat for a few minutes or spread over a baking tray and bake for a couple of minutes. They will cook more evenly in the oven, but keep an eye on them!

NUTRITION (PER SERVE)

CALS	FAT	SAT FAT	PROTEIN	CARBS
340	10g	2g	34g	23g

● EASY   ○ QUICK   ○ MAKE AHEAD   ○ MEAT FREE   ● FAMILY FRIENDLY

★★★★★
Delicious, healthy dinner and is a favourite in our house.
I like to add some baby spinach leaves to the salad.
MUPS6

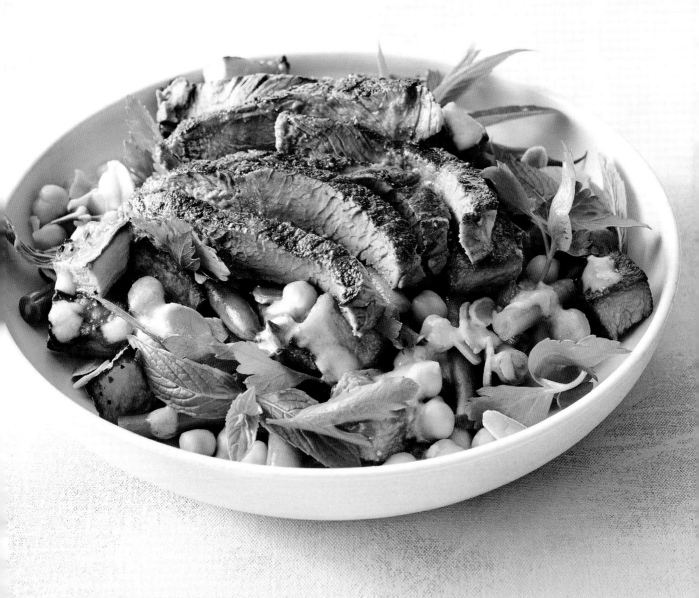

Grilled Vegie
TUNA CARPACCIO

Tuna is a protein powerhouse. Also in there are omega-3 fatty acids and a solid dose of B vitamins, so get grilling!

SERVES 4 **PREP** 15 mins **COOK** 15 mins

350g tomato medley mix, halved if large
¼ cup chopped fresh dill
2 tsp finely grated lemon rind
500g piece sashimi-grade tuna
2 tbs fresh lemon juice
1 long fresh red chilli, deseeded, finely chopped
1 tbs baby capers, rinsed, drained
1 tbs extra virgin olive oil
2 zucchini, thinly sliced lengthways
2 bunches asparagus, trimmed
½ cup small fresh basil leaves

1 Preheat oven to 160°C/140°C fan forced. Line a baking tray with baking paper.
2 Place the tomato on prepared tray and spray lightly with extra virgin olive oil. Roast for 15 minutes or until softened.
3 Meanwhile, combine the dill, lemon rind and a pinch of salt on a plate. Roll the tuna in the dill mixture to coat. Combine the lemon juice, chilli, capers and oil in a small bowl.
4 Heat a barbecue grill or chargrill pan on high. Spray the zucchini, asparagus and tuna with oil. Cook the zucchini and asparagus for 2 minutes each side or until lightly charred and just tender. Cook the tuna for about 1 minute each side or until seared all over. Thinly slice the tuna.
5 Arrange the zucchini, asparagus, tomato and basil on serving plates. Top with the sliced tuna and drizzle over the dressing to serve.

COOK'S NOTE

'Sashimi-grade' means this is the highest-quality tuna and is perfectly safe to eat raw or just seared. Look for it at reputable fishmongers. Serve with wholegrain sourdough, if you like.

NUTRITION (PER SERVE)

CALS	FAT	SAT FAT	PROTEIN	CARBS
270	10g	2g	37g	5g

★★★★★

This was such a beautiful plate of food. Loved the dill coating on the tuna.
DANI.BROUGHAM

● EASY ● QUICK ○ MAKE AHEAD ○ MEAT FREE ○ FAMILY FRIENDLY

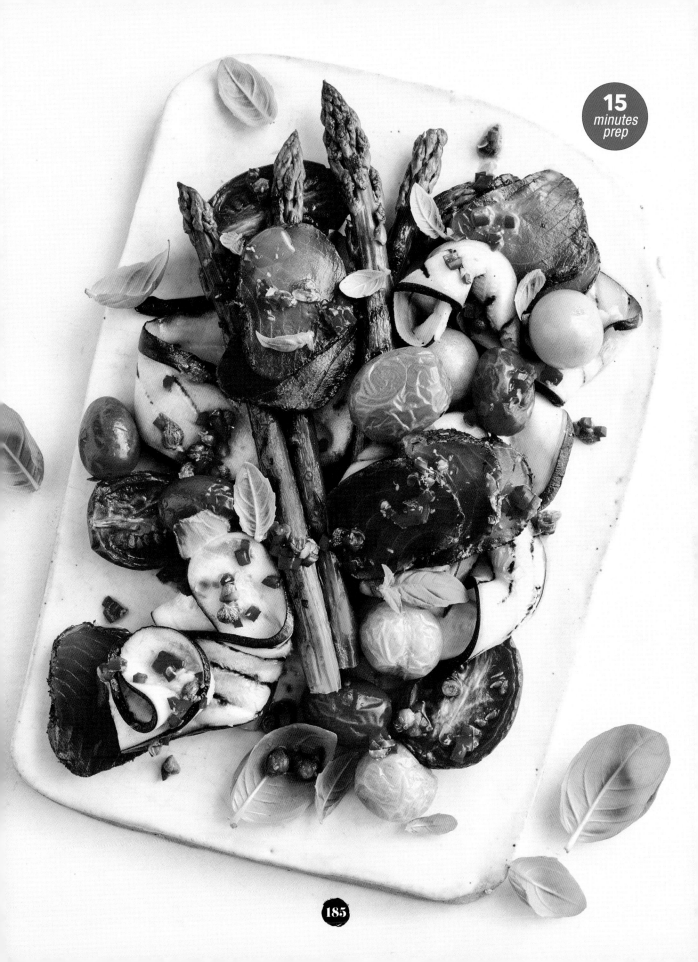

Gremolata - Topped Lentil
BOLOGNAISE

We've given traditional spaghetti bolognaise the veg treatment with mushies and eggplant. Plus, there are zesty lemon gremolata and lentils to boot.

SERVES 6 **PREP** 15 mins **COOK** 30 mins

2 tbs extra virgin olive oil
1 brown onion, finely chopped
1 carrot, peeled, finely chopped
1 celery stick, finely chopped
2 garlic cloves, crushed
200g Swiss brown mushrooms,
  chopped
1 medium eggplant, cut into
  1cm pieces
2 tbs tomato paste
400g can diced tomatoes
250ml (1 cup) vegetable stock
2 tsp Italian dried mixed herbs
3 tsp balsamic vinegar
2 tsp honey
400g can brown lentils,
  rinsed, drained
Cooked spaghetti, to serve
Finely shredded parmesan,
  to serve (optional)
CHILLI GREMOLATA
¼ cup finely chopped fresh
  continental parsley leaves
1 lemon, rind finely grated
Small pinch of dried chilli flakes,
  or to taste

1 Heat the oil in a large deep frying pan over medium-low heat. Add the onion, carrot and celery. Cook, stirring often, for 10 minutes or until soft and lightly coloured. Add the garlic and stir for 1 minute or until aromatic. Add the mushroom and eggplant. Cook, stirring occasionally, for 5 minutes or until softened.
2 Add the tomato paste and stir to coat. Stir in the tomatoes, stock and Italian herbs. Cover and bring to a simmer. Cook for 10 minutes or until thickened slightly. Stir in the vinegar and honey. Add the lentils and stir until heated through. Season.
3 To make the chilli gremolata, combine all the gremolata ingredients in a small bowl.
4 Serve the bolognaise with spaghetti, sprinkled with the gremolata and parmesan, if using.

COOK'S NOTE

The bolognaise sauce can be made ahead. Keep in the fridge for up to 4 days or freeze in airtight containers for up to 1 month.

NUTRITION (PER SERVE)

CALS	FAT	SAT FAT	PROTEIN	CARBS
450	8g	1g	16g	71.5g

● EASY   ○ QUICK   ● MAKE AHEAD   ● MEAT FREE   ○ FAMILY FRIENDLY

15 minutes prep

★ ★ ★ ★ ★

Delicious! Even my meat-eating husband loved it. I made the recipe exactly as stated, but served the sauce with zucchini noodles. I'll make it again for the vegans in the family. **DEB LOWE**

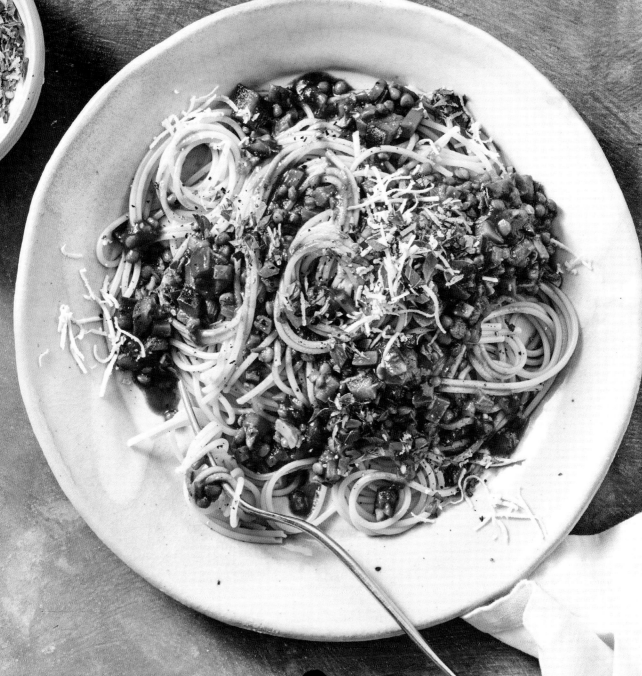

Harissa Chicken
TRAY BAKE

Packed with nourishing ingredients, this tray bake has more than three serves of veg per person and plenty of protein thanks to chicken and lentils.

SERVES 4 **PREP** 25 mins **COOK** 35 mins

3 small carrots, peeled, diagonally sliced

2 large red onions, cut into thin wedges

1 tbs chopped fresh rosemary leaves

1 tbs extra virgin olive oil

2 tsp harissa paste

1 tbs fresh lemon juice (see note)

1 garlic clove, crushed

8 (about 500g) chicken tenderloins, trimmed

400g can no-added-salt brown lentils, rinsed, drained

80g chopped kale leaves

160ml (⅔ cup) salt-reduced chicken stock

90g (⅓ cup) labneh, drained (see note)

Lemon rind cut into thin strips, to serve

1 Preheat oven to 200°C/180°C fan forced. Line a large baking dish or tray with baking paper.

2 Place the carrot, onion and rosemary in prepared dish and drizzle over the oil. Roast for 15-20 minutes or until light golden and tender.

3 Meanwhile, combine the harissa, lemon juice and garlic in a shallow dish. Add the chicken and turn to coat. Set aside for 10 minutes to marinate.

4 Place the lentils, kale and stock in the dish with the carrot mixture and stir to combine. Top with the chicken. Roast for a further 10-15 minutes or until the chicken is cooked through.

5 Top with the labneh and lemon rind. Season and serve.

NUTRITION (PER SERVE)

CALS	FAT	SAT FAT	PROTEIN	CARBS
341	9.5g	2.5g	37.5g	20g

COOK'S NOTE

Cut the rind off the lemon (for garnish) before you juice – much easier to do in this order. Find labneh at specialty food shops or green grocers. Or make your own – check out our recipe on p82. Serve this tray bake with wholemeal pita bread, if you like.

★★★★★

Such an easy, healthy and delicious meal!
Will be making this on repeat :) **CLAIREMcNAB**

● EASY ○ QUICK ○ MAKE AHEAD ○ MEAT FREE ○ FAMILY FRIENDLY

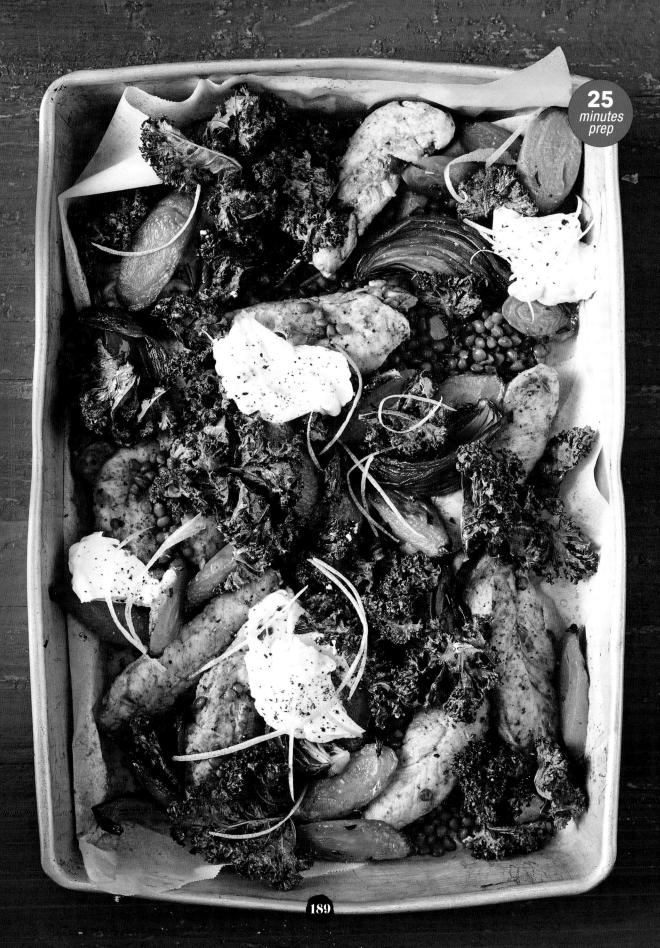

25
*minutes
prep*

189

Spicy Broccolini PRAWN PASTA

Use spelt or wholemeal pasta in place of regular pasta for more fibre and protein. Top it with broccolini – it's known for its cancer-fighting compounds.

SERVES 4 **PREP** 15 mins **COOK** 20 mins

200g dried spelt spaghetti
1 tbs extra virgin olive oil
300g peeled green prawns, deveined, tails intact (see note)
4 garlic cloves, thinly sliced
1 lemon, rind finely grated (see note)
2 long fresh red chillies, deseeded, thinly sliced
2 bunches broccolini, trimmed, cut into 4cm lengths
1 zucchini, halved, thinly sliced
250g cherry tomatoes, halved
1 tbs fresh lemon juice
40g Greek feta, crumbled
½ cup small fresh basil leaves

1 Cook the pasta in a large saucepan of lightly salted boiling water following packet directions or until al dente. Drain. Return to the pan.

2 Meanwhile, heat 1 tsp oil in a large frying pan over high heat. Add the prawns and cook, stirring occasionally, for 3-4 minutes or until golden. Transfer to a plate.

3 Heat 1 tsp of remaining oil in the frying pan over medium heat. Add the garlic, lemon rind and chilli. Cook, stirring, for 1 minute or until aromatic. Add the broccolini, zucchini and 2 tbs water. Cover. Cook for 1 minute or until almost tender. Add the prawns and tomato. Cook, stirring occasionally, for 2 minutes or until the tomato collapses slightly.

4 Add the pasta, lemon juice and remaining 2 tsp oil to the prawn mixture. Toss over medium heat for 1-2 minutes or until well combined and heated through. Divide among serving plates. Sprinkle with the feta and basil to serve.

COOK'S NOTE

Tails on the prawns look good for presentation, but feel free to take them off before cooking, if you like. Use the lemon that you've grated for the 1 tbs juice.

NUTRITION (PER SERVE)

CALS	FAT	SAT FAT	PROTEIN	CARBS
379	9g	2g	28g	40g

★★★★★

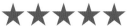

The 'sauce' took no time at all. So many good bits!

FANCY FOODIE

● EASY ○ QUICK ○ MAKE AHEAD ○ MEAT FREE ○ FAMILY FRIENDLY

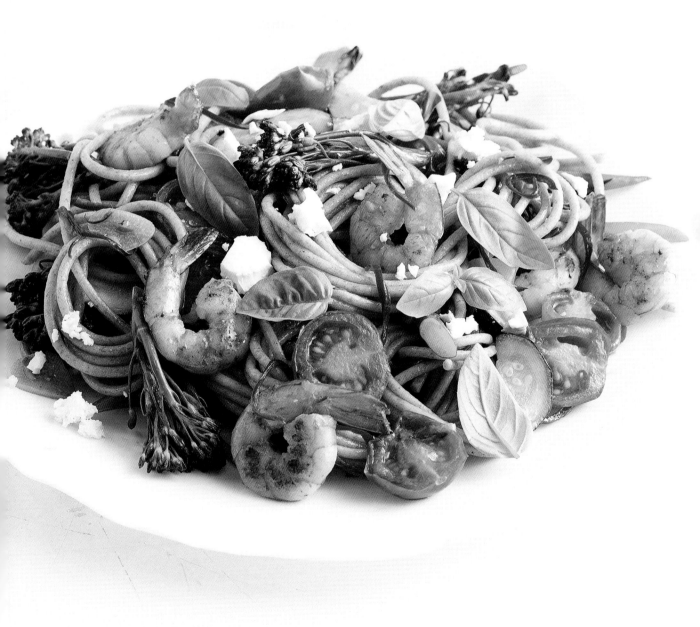

Slow Cooker
FREEKEH BOWL

With only 5 minutes of prep, throw this together in the late afternoon then get on with other things while dinner cooks itself!

SERVES 6 **PREP** 5 mins **COOK** 1 hour 45 mins

1 tbs extra virgin olive oil
1 brown onion, finely chopped
180g (1 cup) freekeh, rinsed, drained
1 tsp ground cinnamon
2 tbs currants
750ml (3 cups) vegetable stock
1 bunch English spinach
1 tbs fresh lemon juice
2 tbs pine nuts, toasted

1 Heat the oil in a large frying pan over medium heat. Add the onion and cook, stirring, for 5 minutes or until softened.
2 Transfer the onion to a slow cooker. Add the freekeh, cinnamon, currants and stock. Cover and cook on High for 1 hour 45 minutes or until tender and most of the stock is absorbed.
3 Stir in the spinach and lemon juice. Set aside for 30 seconds or until the spinach wilts. Season. Divide among serving bowls. Serve sprinkled with the pine nuts.

COOK'S NOTE

Does your slow cooker have the Browning or Saute function? If so, you can make this all in one appliance!

NUTRITION (PER SERVE)

CALS	FAT	SAT FAT	PROTEIN	CARBS
228	9.5g	1.7g	4.2g	30.3g

★★★★★

The freekeh absorbed all of the liquid and the cinnamon and stock gave it a lovely flavour. Kids wanted seconds, so I'll be doubling the quantity next time. **SARAHALLI**

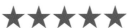

● EASY　○ QUICK　● MAKE AHEAD　● MEAT FREE　● FAMILY FRIENDLY

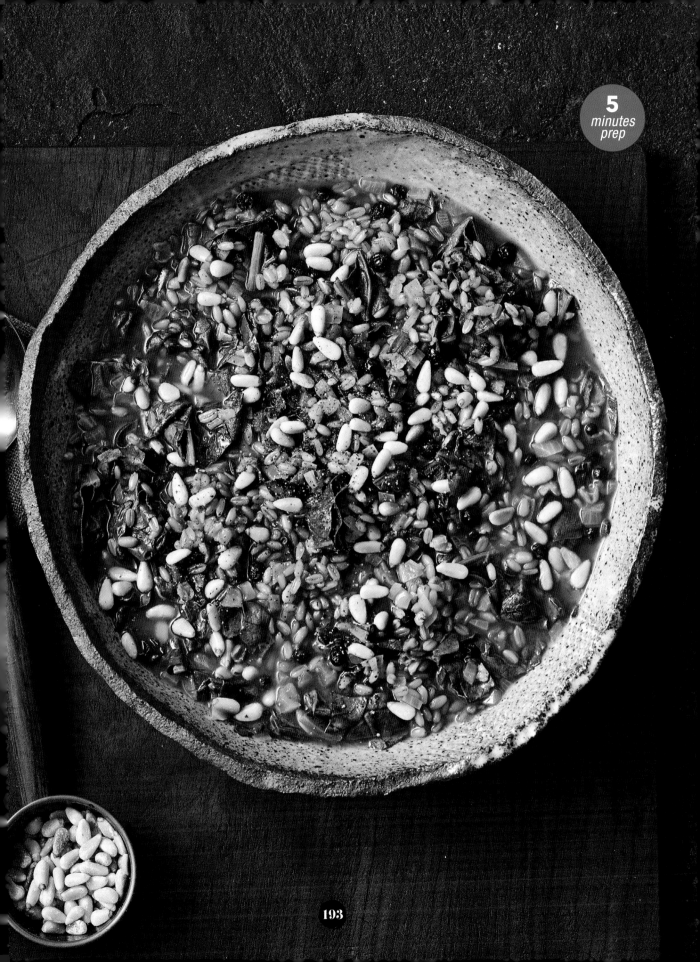

Buckwheat Tabouli with
DUKKAH LAMB

This herby buckwheat salad is really enhanced by the dukkah-crusted lamb on top. We've used backstraps as they're very lean, but oh-so tender.

SERVES 4 **PREP** 10 mins **COOK** 10 mins

150g (¾ cup) buckwheat, rinsed, drained
1 garlic clove, crushed
1 lemon, rind finely grated, juiced
2 tbs extra virgin olive oil
1 tbs white balsamic vinegar
2 (about 480g) lamb backstraps
2 tbs dukkah
3 cups firmly packed fresh mixed herb leaves (such as mint, coriander and parsley)
200g cherry tomatoes, quartered
½ small red onion, finely chopped

1 Bring a saucepan of water to the boil over high heat. Add the buckwheat. Reduce heat to medium-low and simmer for 5-6 minutes or until al dente. Drain and refresh under cold running water. Spread over a tray lined with paper towel to dry.

2 Meanwhile, place the garlic, lemon rind and juice, oil and vinegar in a jar. Season. Seal and shake to combine. Heat a non-stick frying pan over medium heat. Spray the lamb with extra virgin olive oil then season. Cook, turning, for 6-8 minutes for medium or until cooked to your liking. Transfer to a plate. Set aside for 4 minutes to rest.

3 Spread the dukkah over a plate. Press the lamb into the dukkah to coat then slice the lamb.

4 Finely chop three-quarters of the herbs. Place the buckwheat, all the herbs, tomato, onion and half the dressing in a large bowl. Toss to combine. Transfer to a serving platter. Top with the lamb slices. Drizzle over the remaining dressing to serve.

COOK'S NOTE

Dukkah is packed full of flavour. Try sprinkling it over labne or hummus for a tasty dip, on grilled chicken or over salad for extra crunch.

NUTRITION (PER SERVE)

CALS	FAT	SAT FAT	PROTEIN	CARBS
464	18g	4g	41g	29g

● EASY ● QUICK ○ MAKE AHEAD ○ MEAT FREE ● FAMILY FRIENDLY

★ ★ ★ ★ ★

Love finding new ways to twist meat and three veg!

WAFFLEISO

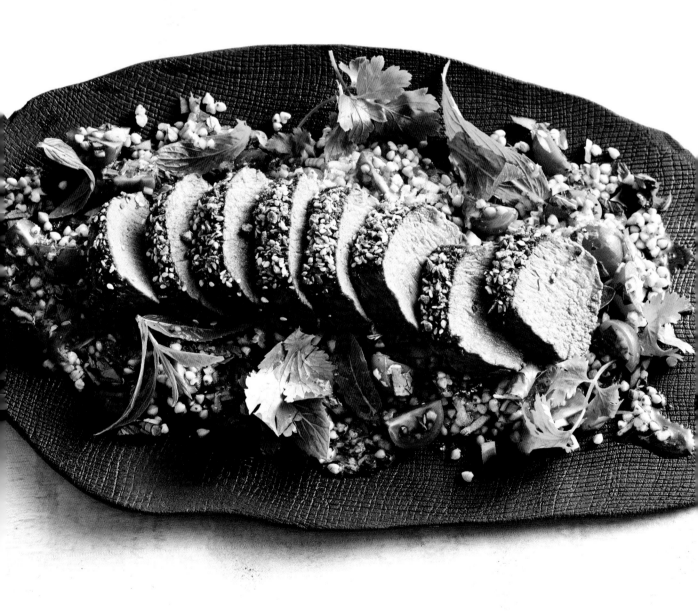

Cannellini & Tomato
ONE-PAN FISH

Got 20 minutes? That's all you need to fry up this fish dish! The cannellini are a budget way to get more of the nutrients embraced by the Mediterranean diet.

SERVES 4 **PREP** 5 mins **COOK** 15 mins

4 (150g each) thick white fish fillets (see note)
1 tbs extra virgin olive oil
2 small leeks, thinly sliced
2 garlic cloves, crushed
1 tbs pine nuts
1 tbs baby capers, drained
200g small cherry tomatoes
400g can cannellini beans, rinsed, drained
50g baby spinach
1-2 tbs fresh lemon juice, to taste
Lemon wedges, to serve

1 Season the fish. Heat half the oil in a large non-stick frying pan over medium-high heat. Cook the fish for 2-3 minutes each side or until golden and cooked through. Transfer to a plate and cover to keep warm.

2 Add the remaining oil to the pan. Cook the leek for 1-2 minutes or until just softened. Add the garlic and pine nuts. Cook for 1 minute or until light golden. Add the capers and tomatoes. Cook, stirring often, for 3-4 minutes or until the tomatoes begin to collapse.

3 Add the cannellini beans and spinach. Cook, stirring, until the spinach wilts. Pour in the lemon juice and season well. Return the fish to the pan and heat until heated through. Serve with lemon wedges to squeeze over.

COOK'S NOTE

Use any thick white-fleshed fish, such as ling, blue-eye trevalla, coral trout, John Dory or bream.

NUTRITION (PER SERVE)

CALS	FAT	SAT FAT	PROTEIN	CARBS
299	10g	1.5g	35.5g	12g

★★★★★

I so enjoyed this meal! I am a non-seafood person, but this will now be a regular in my meal planning!

LIZH

● EASY ● QUICK ○ MAKE AHEAD ○ MEAT FREE ● FAMILY FRIENDLY

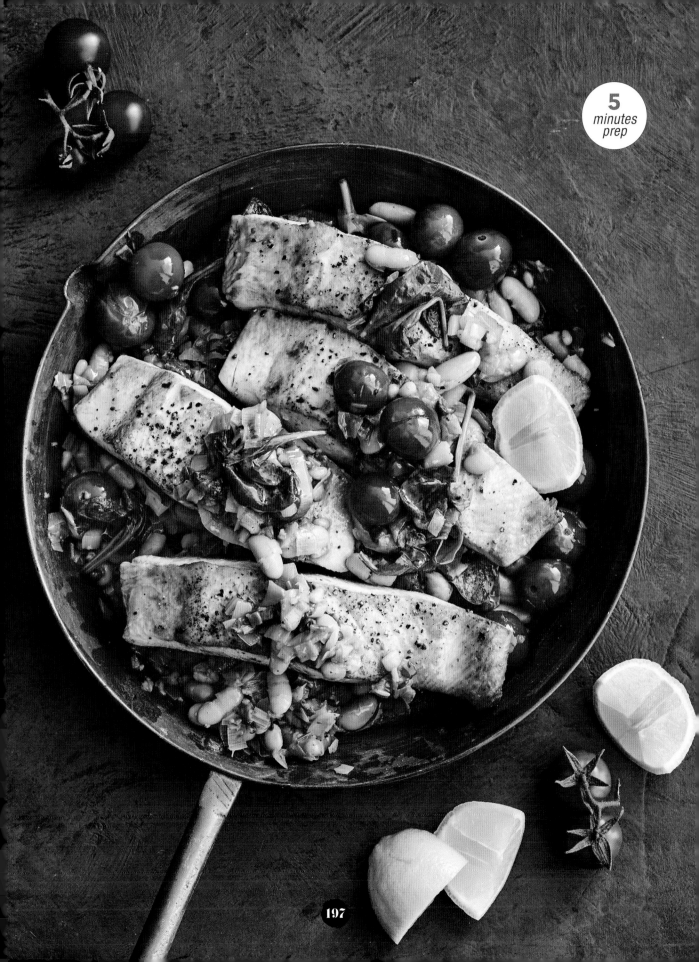

5
minutes
prep

Cauliflower & Salmon
PASTA BAKE

This is a great one to have in the line up for busy weeknights. If your pantry is stocked with canned salmon and tomatoes, you're halfway there!

SERVES 6 **PREP** 15 mins **COOK** 25 mins

300g wholemeal dried penne pasta
500g cauliflower, cut into florets
1 tbs extra virgin olive oil
1 brown onion, finely chopped
2 large garlic cloves, crushed
2 x 400g cans cherry tomatoes
2 tsp balsamic vinegar
415g can red salmon, drained, flaked
60g baby spinach
100g fresh ricotta, crumbled
30g finely shredded parmesan
Small fresh basil leaves, to serve

1 Preheat oven to 200°C/180°C fan forced.
2 Cook the pasta in a large saucepan of lightly salted boiling water for 7 minutes, adding the cauliflower in the last 3 minutes of cooking. Drain well.
3 Meanwhile, heat the oil in a large deep frying pan over medium heat. Add the onion and cook, stirring, for 5 minutes or until soft. Add the garlic and cook, stirring, for 30 seconds. Add the tomatoes and vinegar. Season.
4 Combine the tomato mixture, pasta, cauliflower, salmon and spinach in a 3L (12 cup) baking dish. Dot with the ricotta and sprinkle with the parmesan. Season. Bake for 15 minutes or until the cheese is melted. Sprinkle with basil to serve.

COOK'S NOTE

Swap the salmon for canned tuna, if you prefer. For a vego version, saute thickly sliced mushrooms with the onion.

NUTRITION (PER SERVE)

CALS	FAT	SAT FAT	PROTEIN	CARBS
383	12g	3.7g	24g	41g

★★★★★

This is fantastic, easy, tasty, really quick to whip up for an easy dinner. Excellent dish.

VICKTHECHICK

● EASY ○ QUICK ○ MAKE AHEAD ○ MEAT FREE ● FAMILY FRIENDLY

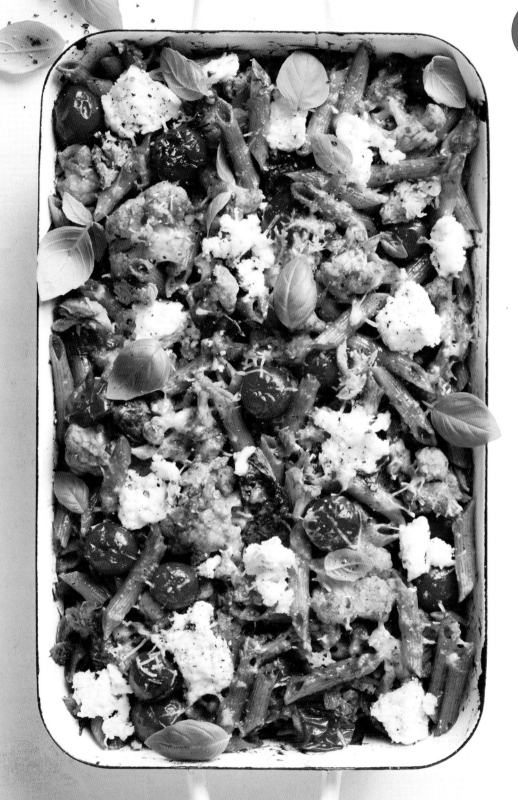

Spicy Bean & Olive
SPANISH CHICKEN

Want to get ahead with meal prep? You can freeze the elements of this super veg, lean chicken winner to make busy dinnertime a breeze.

SERVES 4 **PREP** 10 mins **COOK** 15 mins

2 tsp smoked paprika
2 tsp harissa paste
4 garlic cloves, thinly sliced
2 tbs fresh lemon juice
8 (about 500g) chicken tenderloins
250g green beans, chopped
2 x 400g cans no-added-salt
   cannellini beans, rinsed, drained
2 small zucchini, sliced
85g (½ cup) pitted Sicilian
   green olives, halved
2 x 400g cans cherry tomatoes
2 tsp extra virgin olive oil
Fresh continental parsley sprigs,
   to serve

1 Combine the paprika, harissa, garlic and lemon juice in a large bowl. Add the chicken and turn to coat.
2 Place the green beans, cannellini beans, zucchini, olives and tomatoes in a separate large bowl. Toss until combined.
3 Heat the oil in a large frying pan. Add the chicken mixture. Cook for 2 minutes each side or until browned. Add the bean mixture and simmer for 10 minutes or until the vegetables are just tender. Divide among serving plates. Top with parsley to serve.

NUTRITION (PER SERVE)

CALS	FAT	SAT FAT	PROTEIN	CARBS
368	11g	2g	41g	23g

COOK'S NOTE

This will keep in the freezer for up to 3 months. Do step 1 in an airtight container and step 2 in another container. Freeze both. Defrost overnight in the fridge then continue with step 3. Serve with steamed wholemeal couscous or quinoa, if you like.

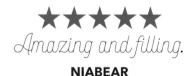

★★★★★
Amazing and filling.
NIABEAR

● EASY ● QUICK ● MAKE AHEAD ○ MEAT FREE ○ FAMILY FRIENDLY

10 minutes prep

★ ★ ★ ★ ★

Yummo! Easy, delicious recipe.

SHIRLEEN

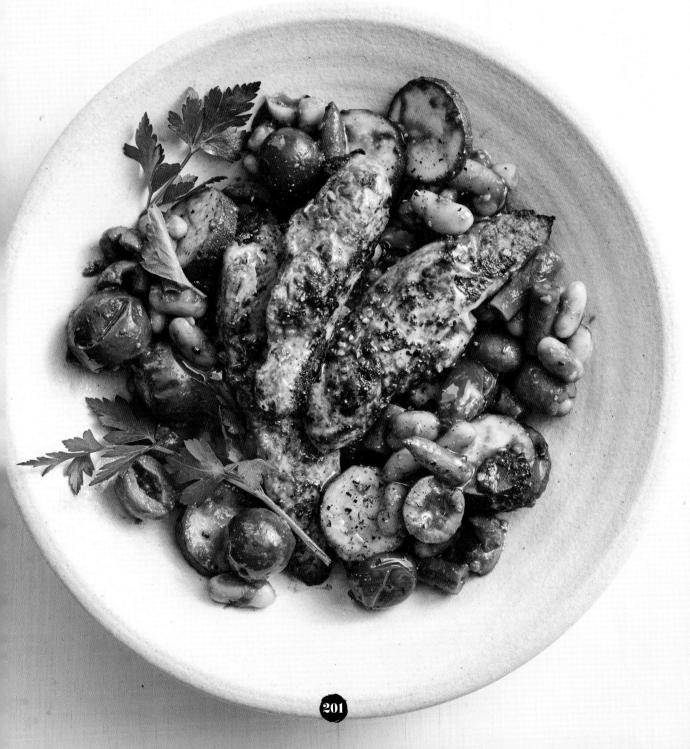

Mackerel & Basil FISH CAKES

If you love fish and chips, then you'll love this modern, better-for-you twist. Leave the battered variety behind for panko-crumbed fish cakes with salad.

SERVES 4 **PREP** 20 mins (+ cooling & 20 mins chilling) **COOK** 25 mins

800g desiree potatoes, peeled, chopped
2 x 115g cans skinless and boneless mackerel fillets, drained
3 green shallots, finely chopped
½ cup chopped fresh basil leaves
2 tbs sliced kalamata olives
1 tsp finely grated lemon rind
1 egg, lightly whisked
70g (1⅓ cups) panko breadcrumbs
Extra virgin olive oil, to shallow fry
Lemon wedges, to serve

TOMATO AND CANNELLINI BEAN SALAD
200g grape tomatoes, halved
400g can cannellini beans, rinsed, drained
2 tsp finely chopped fresh oregano leaves
1 gem lettuce, leaves separated
2 tbs balsamic vinegar dressing

1 Place the potato in a large saucepan and cover with plenty of cold water. Bring to the boil over high heat. Boil for 12 minutes or until tender. Drain the potato then return to the pan over low heat. Toss until the liquid has evaporated. Coarsely mash. Transfer to a bowl. Set aside to cool slightly.
2 Add the mackerel, shallot, basil, olives, lemon rind, egg and 20g (⅓ cup) breadcrumbs to the potato. Season. Stir until combined. Use damp hands to shape the mixture into 8 patties.
3 Place the remaining breadcrumbs in a shallow dish. Coat the patties in the breadcrumbs, shaking off the excess. Place on a plate lined with baking paper. Place in the fridge for 20 minutes or until firm.
4 Meanwhile, make the tomato and cannellini bean salad. Combine the tomato, cannellini beans, oregano and lettuce in a bowl. Drizzle over the dressing. Season and toss gently until combined.
5 Add oil to a large non-stick frying pan to come 1cm up the side of the pan. Heat over medium heat. Shallow-fry the patties for 2 minutes each side or until golden and crisp. Drain on paper towel. Serve the patties with the salad and lemon wedges to squeeze over.

COOK'S NOTE

Patties can be made ahead and frozen for up to 2 months. Wrap each one tightly in foil then place in an airtight freezer bag. Thaw in the fridge overnight.

NUTRITION (PER SERVE)

CALS	FAT	SAT FAT	PROTEIN	CARBS
666	33.1g	6.9g	26g	63.3g

○ EASY   ○ QUICK   ● MAKE AHEAD   ○ MEAT FREE   ● FAMILY FRIENDLY

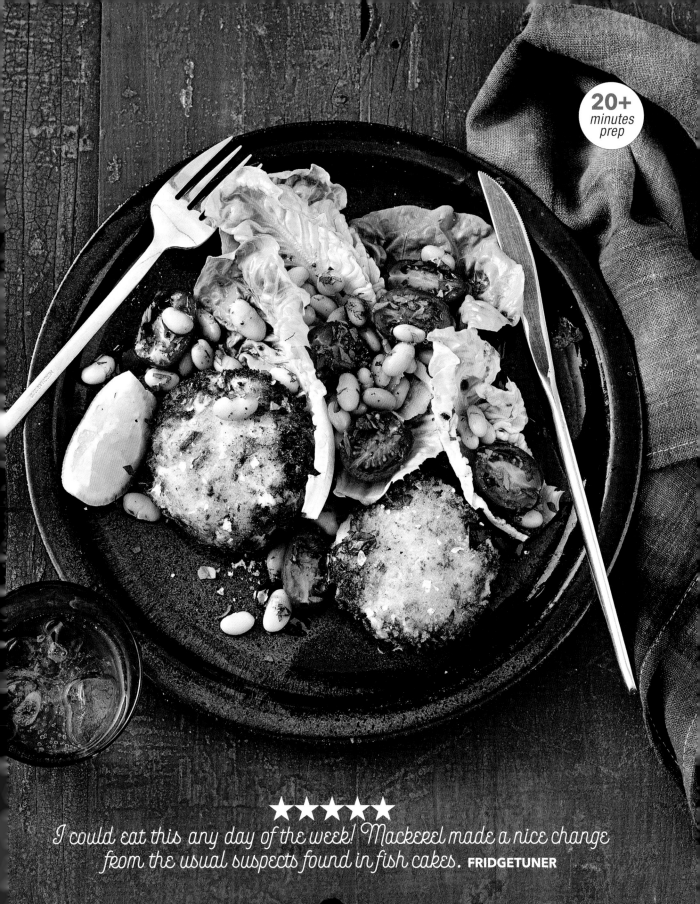

★★★★★

I could eat this any day of the week! Mackerel made a nice change from the usual suspects found in fish cakes. **FRIDGETUNER**

Sweet Potato
BLACK BEAN BOWL

Sweet potato sliced and roasted makes moreish chips that fill you up. Let them get nice and crispy while this spiced vegie mix bubbles away.

SERVES 4 **PREP** 20 mins **COOK** 25 mins

600g sweet potato, peeled,
  thinly sliced
2 tsp ground cumin
2 tsp smoked paprika
2 tsp extra virgin olive oil
2 garlic cloves, crushed
400g can black beans,
  rinsed, drained
1 large zucchini, finely chopped
150g green beans, cut into
  2cm lengths
1 corncob, kernels removed
3 vine ripened tomatoes,
  finely chopped
90g (⅓ cup) Greek-style yoghurt
1 red onion, finely chopped
Fresh coriander sprigs, to serve

1 Preheat oven to 200°C/180°C fan forced. Line 2 large baking trays with baking paper.
2 Place the sweet potato in a single layer on prepared trays. Lightly spray with extra virgin olive oil. Combine the cumin and paprika in a bowl. Sprinkle the sweet potato with half the spice mixture. Roast, swapping trays halfway through cooking, for 25-30 minutes or until golden and slightly crisp.
3 Meanwhile, heat the oil in a large deep non-stick frying pan over medium heat. Add the garlic and remaining spice mixture. Cook, stirring, for 1 minute or until aromatic. Add the black beans. Cook, stirring, for 2 minutes. Add the zucchini, green beans and corn. Cook, stirring, for 2 minutes. Add the tomato and simmer for 5 minutes or until the vegetables are tender.
4 Divide the sweet potato chips and bean mixture among serving bowls. Top with the yoghurt, onion and coriander. Season and serve.

COOK'S NOTE

Don't have black beans in the pantry? Canned chickpeas or kidney beans would work just as well.

NUTRITION (PER SERVE)

CALS	FAT	SAT FAT	PROTEIN	CARBS
323	7.5g	1.6g	13.4g	45.4g

★★★★★

A little bit out there for our normal meals, but was pleasantly surprised, more filling than expected. Would have it again. **DARLYP**

● EASY ○ QUICK ○ MAKE AHEAD ● MEAT FREE ● FAMILY FRIENDLY

20
minutes
prep

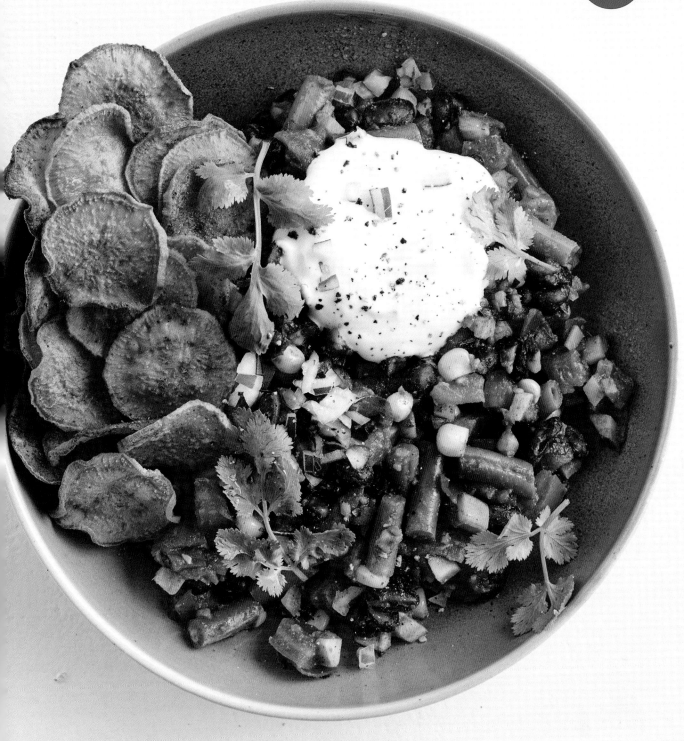

Honey & Lentil BARRA TRAY BAKE

Top tender barramundi fillets and caramelised veg with a zesty carrot top gremolata. Sweet, smoky and tangy, this dish only takes 10 minutes to prep!

SERVES 4 **PREP** 10 mins **COOK** 35 mins

1 bunch baby carrots, scrubbed, trimmed, fronds reserved
1 red onion, unpeeled, cut into wedges
1 lemon, quartered
125ml (½ cup) extra virgin olive oil
1 tbs honey
1 tbs harissa
4 (130g each) barramundi fillets, skin on
1 garlic clove, crushed
1 tbs fresh lemon juice
400g can brown lentils, rinsed, drained
1 bunch asparagus, trimmed

1 Preheat oven to 220°C/200°C fan forced.
2 Place the carrots, onion and lemon on a large baking tray. Drizzle over 1 tbs oil. Season and toss to coat. Roast for 20 minutes or until softened and light golden.
3 Meanwhile, combine the honey and harissa in a bowl. Add the barramundi and turn to coat.
4 Place the garlic, reserved carrot fronds, lemon juice and 60ml (¼ cup) of the remaining oil in a small food processor. Process until almost smooth. Season then transfer the gremolata to a small serving bowl.
5 Add the barramundi, lentils and asparagus to the tray. Drizzle over the remaining oil. Roast for 15 minutes or until the barramundi flesh flakes easily when tested with a fork in the thickest part. Drizzle some of the gremolata over the tray bake. Season then serve with the remaining gremolata on the side.

COOK'S NOTE

A bunch of baby carrots is a great use-it-all veg! Hold on to the fronds – their earthiness is delicious in salads, or blitzed into pesto, hummus or smoothies. Just be sure to wash them well.

NUTRITION (PER SERVE)

CALS	FAT	SAT FAT	PROTEIN	CARBS
549	36.8g	6.1g	32.7g	21.3g

★★★★★

Easy, quick and so fresh! Absolutely loved this one, would definitely recommend going to the effort to make the gremolata. **GL**

● **EASY** ○ QUICK ○ MAKE AHEAD ○ MEAT FREE ○ FAMILY FRIENDLY

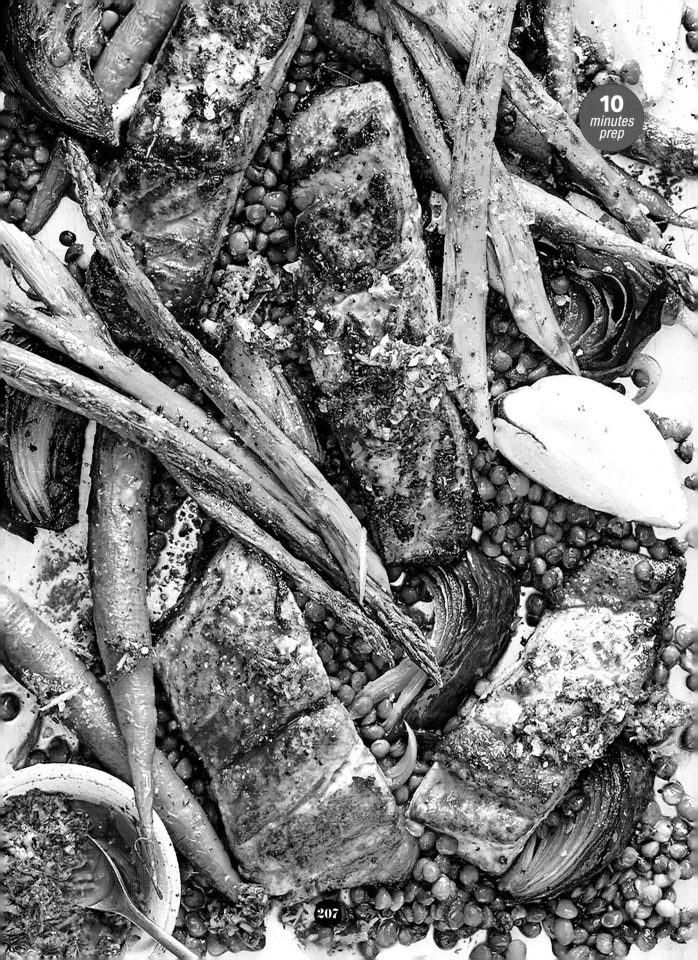

Zesty Grilled
GARLIC CHICKEN

These lean chicken tenderloins are marinated in lemon, lime and garlic.
Team them with broccolini, lightly cooked to preserve its nutrients.

SERVES 4 **PREP** 15 mins (+ 30 mins marinating) **COOK** 15 mins

2 tsp finely grated lemon rind,
  plus extra to serve
1 tsp finely grated lime rind
1½ tbs fresh lemon juice
3 garlic cloves, crushed
3 tsp extra virgin olive oil
8 large (about 500g) chicken
  tenderloins
1 red onion, finely chopped
2 celery sticks, thinly sliced
2 bunches broccolini, trimmed,
  cut into 5cm lengths
400g can chickpeas, rinsed, drained
100g baby kale leaves
40g Greek feta, crumbled

1 Combine the lemon and lime rind, lemon juice, one-third of the garlic and 2 tsp oil in a shallow dish. Add the chicken and turn to coat. Cover and place in the fridge for 30 minutes to marinate.
2 Preheat a barbecue grill or chargrill pan on medium-high. Grill the chicken for 2 minutes each side or until lightly charred and cooked through.
3 Meanwhile, heat the remaining oil in a large saucepan over medium heat. Add the onion and celery. Cook, stirring, for 5 minutes. Add the remaining garlic and cook, stirring, for 30 seconds or until aromatic. Add the broccolini, chickpeas and 2 tbs water. Cover and cook, stirring occasionally, for 2 minutes or until the broccolini is tender crisp. Stir through the kale and cook for 1-2 minutes or until just wilted.
4 Divide the broccolini mixture among serving plates. Top with the chicken. Scatter over the feta and extra lemon rind to serve.

COOK'S NOTE

Don't worry if you're short on time to marinate the chicken. Just put it in the fridge while you prepare the vegies – it will still taste great! Serve with steamed wholemeal couscous or brown rice, if you like.

NUTRITION (PER SERVE)

CALS	FAT	SAT FAT	PROTEIN	CARBS
311	9g	3g	39g	12g

★★★★★

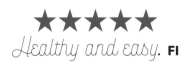

Healthy and easy. **FI**

● EASY ○ QUICK ○ MAKE AHEAD ○ MEAT FREE ● FAMILY FRIENDLY

15+
minutes prep

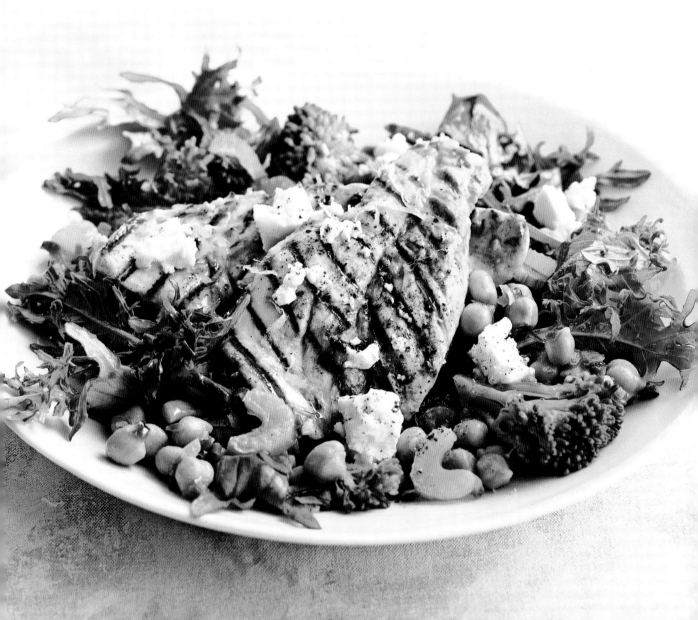

Prep-Ahead
SEAFOOD STEW

A little planning on the weekend goes a long way to making midweek effort minimal. Simply chop the veg, marinate the seafood and freeze.

SERVES 6 **PREP** 20 mins **COOK** 40 mins

4 (150g each) skinless salmon fillets

500g green prawns, peeled, deveined, tails intact

1 lemon, rind finely grated, plus extra rind, cut into thin strips, to serve

1 tbs finely chopped fresh continental parsley leaves

400g can baby roma tomatoes

1 small fennel bulb, finely chopped

1 leek, halved, thinly sliced

1 celery stick, thinly sliced

1 carrot, peeled, finely chopped

2 garlic cloves, sliced

1 long fresh red chilli, finely sliced

2 tbs baby capers, rinsed, drained, plus extra, fried, to serve

4 anchovies, drained, finely chopped

125ml (½ cup) white wine

750ml (3 cups) vegetable stock

Small basil leaves, to serve (optional)

1 Place the salmon, prawns, lemon rind and parsley in a large bowl. Toss to coat.

2 Place the tomatoes, fennel, leek, celery, carrot, garlic, chilli, capers, anchovy, wine and stock in a separate large bowl. Stir until combined.

3 Transfer the tomato mixture to a large heavy-based saucepan. Bring to the boil over medium heat. Reduce heat to low and simmer for 30 minutes or until thickens slightly and vegetables are tender. Add the seafood mixture. Cook for a further 7-10 minutes or until the seafood is cooked through. Top with extra lemon rind, extra fried capers and basil, if using.

NUTRITION (PER SERVE)

CALS	FAT	SAT FAT	PROTEIN	CARBS
316	14.5g	3g	32.8g	7.1g

COOK'S NOTE

This will keep in the freezer for up to 3 months. Do step 1 in an airtight container and step 2 in another container. Freeze both. Defrost overnight in the fridge then continue with step 3. Sere with wholegrain sourdough bread or steamed greens, if you like.

★ ★ ★ ★ ★

I made this and it was loved by all. Yummy.

WENDY SCHMIDT

● EASY   ○ QUICK   ● MAKE AHEAD   ○ MEAT FREE   ○ FAMILY FRIENDLY

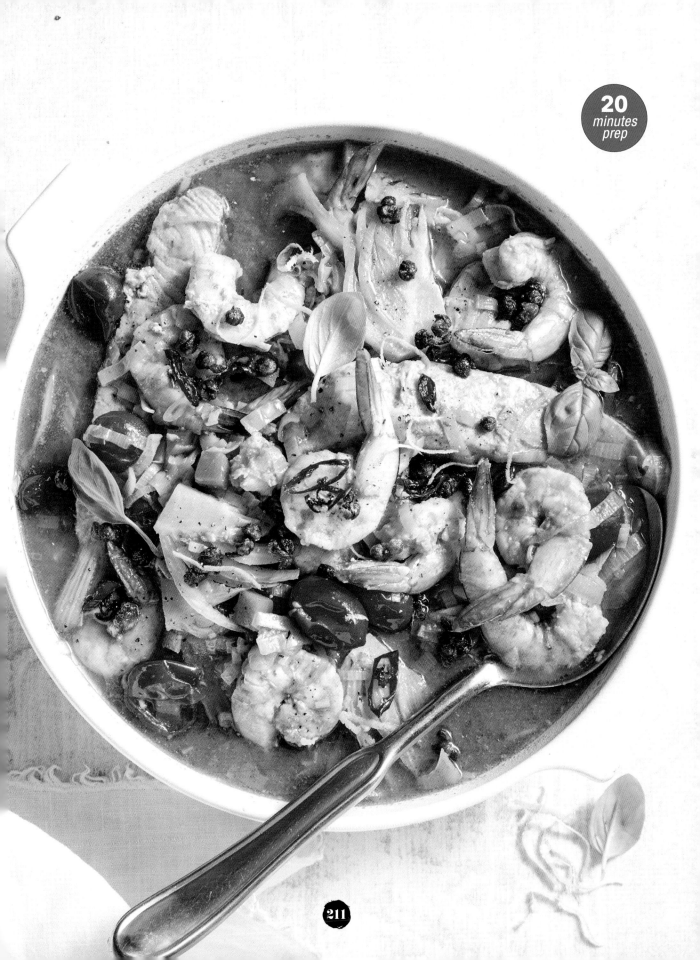

Freekeh & Eggplant
CUMIN LAMB

The Mediterranean diet is a way of life, so enjoy things like red meat in moderation, pick lean cuts and serve with grains and plenty of veg.

SERVES 4 **PREP** 20 mins **COOK** 40 mins

180g (1 cup) freekeh, rinsed, drained
3 tsp ground cumin
2½ tbs extra virgin olive oil
80ml (⅓ cup) fresh lemon juice
2 small eggplants
1 (about 280g) lamb backstrap
1 small red onion, finely chopped
200g tomato medley mix, halved
⅓ cup fresh mint leaves
¼ cup fresh continental
   parsley leaves
2 tbs fresh dill
200g tzatziki (to make your own
   see our recipe on p52)

1 Place the freekeh and 625ml (2½ cups) water in a saucepan over high heat. Bring to the boil then reduce heat to low. Simmer, covered, for 35 minutes or until tender and liquid is absorbed.
2 Meanwhile, combine the cumin, 2 tbs oil and 2 tbs lemon juice in a glass or ceramic dish. Season. Cut the eggplant lengthways into 5mm-thick slices and add to the dish. Rub to coat in the cumin mixture.
3 Heat a barbecue grill or chargrill pan on medium-high. Grill the eggplant for 3 minutes each side or until charred and tender. Transfer to a large bowl. Add the lamb to the dish with the remaining cumin mixture. Toss to coat. Grill the lamb for 5 minutes each side for medium or until cooked to your liking. Transfer to a plate. Cover and set aside for 5 minutes to rest. Slice the lamb then add to the eggplant bowl.
4 Add the freekeh, onion, tomato, mint, parsley, dill and remaining lemon juice to the bowl. Season and toss until combined.
5 Spread the tzatziki over a large serving plate. Top with the eggplant and lamb mixture. Drizzle over the remaining oil, season and serve.

COOK'S NOTE

If freekeh isn't available, use brown rice instead.

NUTRITION (PER SERVE)

CALS	FAT	SAT FAT	PROTEIN	CARBS
521	19.5g	4.4g	36.9g	47.1g

● EASY ○ QUICK ○ MAKE AHEAD ○ MEAT FREE ● FAMILY FRIENDLY

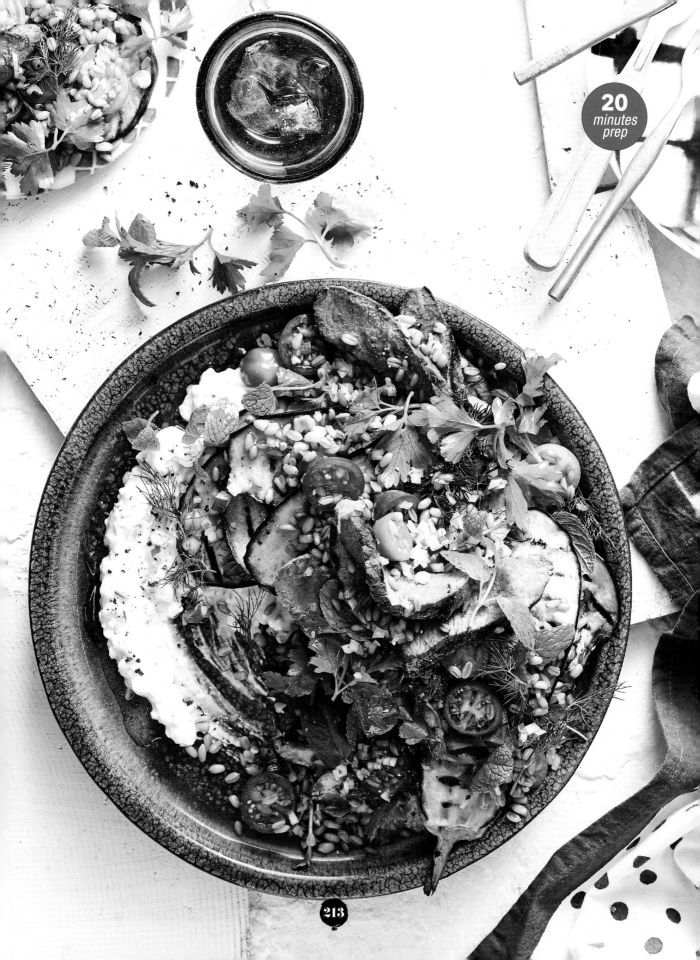

20
minutes
prep

213

Speedy Potato & Olive SALMON BAKE

This quick and easy tray bake ticks the box when it comes to getting a variety of vegies all in one meal.

SERVES 4 **PREP** 5 mins **COOK** 25 mins

8 baby coliban (chat) potatoes,
  cut into 5mm-thick slices
250g cherry tomatoes
2 tsp extra virgin olive oil
4 (150g each) salmon fillets, skin on
50g (¼ cup) kalamata olives
1 tbs baby capers, rinsed, drained
1 lemon, rind finely grated
⅓ cup small fresh basil leaves
Mixed salad leaves, to serve

1 Preheat oven to 200°C/180°C fan forced.
2 Evenly arrange the potato over the base of a large baking dish. Scatter over the cherry tomatoes. Drizzle over the oil then bake for 15 minutes.
3 Arrange the salmon, skin-side down, in the dish. Sprinkle with the olives, capers and lemon rind. Season well. Bake for a further 10 minutes.
4 Scatter over the basil and serve immediately with salad leaves on the side.

COOK'S NOTE

Not sure what to do with a rindless lemon? Squeeze the juice into an ice cube tray and freeze for another use.

NUTRITION (PER SERVE)

CALS	FAT	SAT FAT	PROTEIN	CARBS
480	30.4g	6.3g	33.9g	15.4g

★★★★★

Definitely a winner in our house. Simple to make and very tasty.
MRSGANDIE

● EASY   ● QUICK   ○ MAKE AHEAD   ○ MEAT FREE   ● FAMILY FRIENDLY

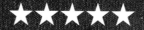

★★★★★

So simple to make and really delicious. The ingredients aren't too fancy, but it looks and tastes like gourmet.

RELUCTANTCOOK

5 minutes prep

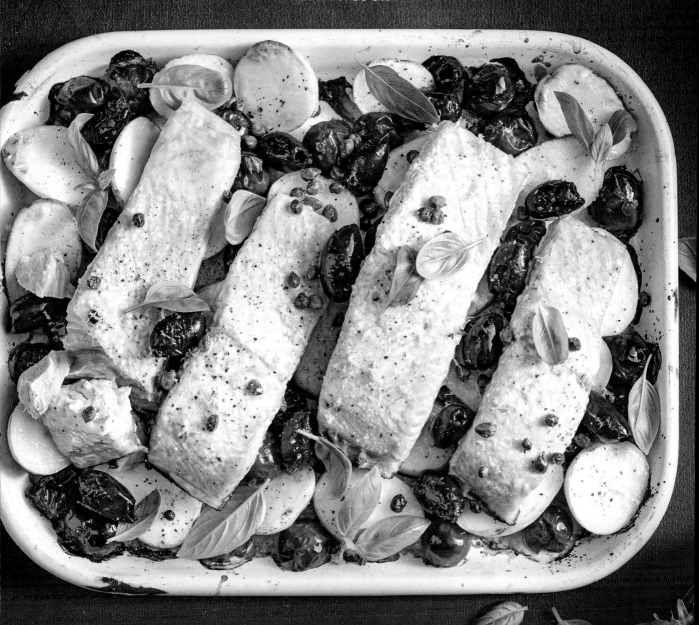

Chicken & Ricotta
ZUCCHINI RAVIOLI

Before you baulk at making ravioli, have a go at this simple, better-for-you twist. Made with thinly sliced zucchini, this is a great way to skip processed pasta.

SERVES 4 **PREP** 15 mins **COOK** 35 mins

100g baby spinach
250g chicken mince
100g fresh ricotta
¼ cup finely chopped fresh
    continental parsley leaves
20g (¼ cup) finely grated parmesan
2 tsp finely grated lemon rind
1 egg yolk
400g can cherry tomatoes
2 garlic cloves, crushed
2 large zucchini, thinly sliced
    lengthways (see note)
55g (½ cup) coarsely grated
    mozzarella
2 tbs pine nuts

1 Preheat oven to 190°C/170°C fan forced. Lightly spray a large baking dish with extra virgin olive oil.
2 Heat a frying pan over high heat. Cook the spinach, stirring, for 3-5 minutes or until wilted. Remove from heat, drain in a sieve and squeeze out any moisture. Finely chop.
3 Combine the spinach, chicken, ricotta, parsley, parmesan, lemon rind and egg yolk in a bowl. Season. Combine the tomatoes and garlic in a separate bowl. Season.
4 Lay 2 zucchini slices, slightly overlapping, on a clean surface. Lay 2 more slices, slightly overlapping, at right angles to form a cross. Shape ¼ cupful of the chicken mixture into a patty. Place in the centre of the cross. Fold the zucchini slices over to form a parcel. Arrange the ravioli, seam-side down, in prepared dish. Repeat with the remaining zucchini slices and chicken mixture to make 8 ravioli in total.
5 Spoon the tomato mixture around the ravioli. Top with the mozzarella and pine nuts. Bake for 30 minutes or until golden and cooked through. Season and serve.

COOK'S NOTE

Thinly slice the zucchini so it doesn't break while folding. Use a mandolin, if you have one. Make this dish up to 1 day ahead (without baking) and chill. Return to room temperature then cook as directed. Serve with wholegrain sourdough bread, if you like.

NUTRITION (PER SERVE)

CALS	FAT	SAT FAT	PROTEIN	CARBS
299	19g	6.5g	23g	6.5g

○ EASY   ○ QUICK   ● MAKE AHEAD   ○ MEAT FREE   ● FAMILY FRIENDLY

15
minutes
prep

★ ★ ★ ★ ★

Delicious. Topped the dish with mozzarella and parmesan.
Loved the pine nuts. **TOOKUSTER**

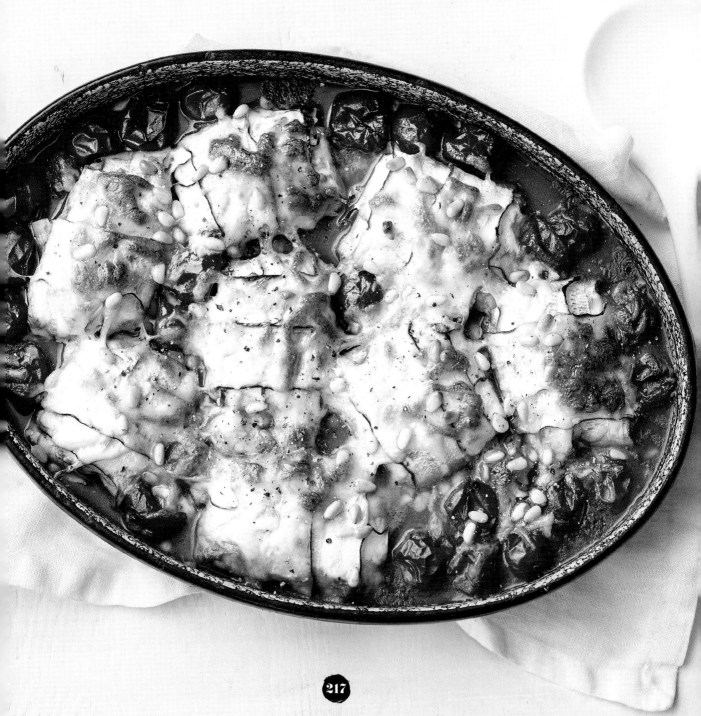

Spicy Baked
FISH CUTLETS

Canned and frozen veg, with a little help from your spice rack, are your simple shortcut to eating more of the ingredients to hit your #MedGoals!

SERVES 4 **PREP** 10 mins **COOK** 15 mins

2 tsp fennel seeds, crushed
1 tsp sweet paprika
½ tsp dried chilli flakes
4 fish cutlets (see note)
2½ tbs extra virgin olive oil,
   plus extra to drizzle
3 garlic cloves, thinly sliced
1 lemon, halved lengthways, sliced
400g can cherry tomatoes
   or diced tomatoes
400g can butter beans,
   rinsed, drained
55g (⅓ cup) pitted kalamata olives
300g frozen broad beans
Wholegrain sourdough bread,
   to serve

1 Preheat oven to 220°C/200°C fan forced.
2 Combine the fennel seeds, paprika and chilli in a small bowl. Season. Rub the fish cutlets all over with 1 tbs oil then sprinkle both sides with the spice mixture.
3 Heat the remaining oil in a large ovenproof frying pan over medium heat. Add the fish and cook for 1 minute 30 seconds each side or until browned but not quite cooked through. Transfer to a plate.
4 Add the garlic to the pan and cook, stirring, for 1 minute or until aromatic. Add the lemon and cook, turning, for 1 minute or until it starts to caramelise. Add the tomatoes, butter beans and olives. Bring to a simmer then arrange the fish on top. Transfer the pan to the oven and bake for 5 minutes.
5 Meanwhile, place the broad beans in a heatproof bowl. Cover with boiling water and set aside for 1 minute. Drain then squeeze the beans from the skins.
6 Gently stir the broad beans into the tomato mixture then bake for a further 5 minutes or until the fish is just cooked through.
7 Drizzle over a little extra oil. Serve with sourdough.

COOK'S NOTE

Go for blue-eye trevalla, salmon or ocean trout. We used cutlets from the tail end because they cook more evenly.

NUTRITION (PER SERVE)

CALS	FAT	SAT FAT	PROTEIN	CARBS
566	21.8g	3.6g	46.6g	39.9g

● EASY ○ QUICK ○ MAKE AHEAD ○ MEAT FREE ○ FAMILY FRIENDLY

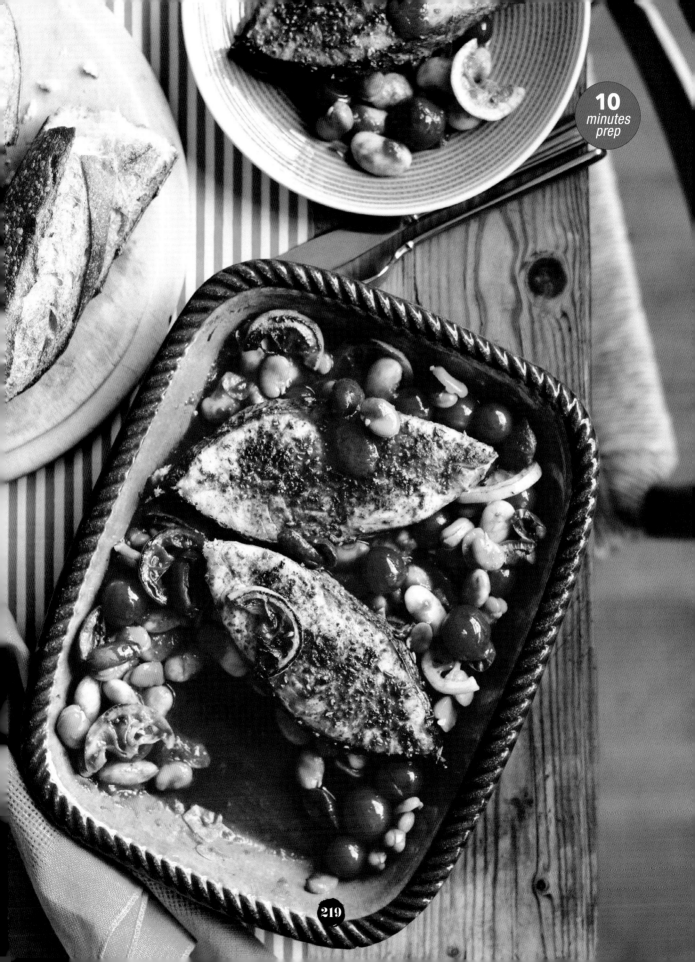

Lentil Salad with
BARBECUED FISH

A fuss-free marinade of lemon, olive oil and dill spruces up white fish.
Grill zucchini and squash, and this quick dinner is ready to go!

SERVES 4 **PREP** 15 mins (+ 10 mins marinating) **COOK** 10 mins

2 tbs fresh lemon juice
1 tbs extra virgin olive oil
2 tbs chopped fresh dill, plus extra, chopped, to serve
4 (125g each) firm white fish fillets
2 large zucchini, cut into 5mm-thick slices
4 yellow squash, cut into 5mm-thick slices
400g can no-added-salt lentils, rinsed, drained
250g tomato medley mix, halved
¼ cup fresh continental parsley leaves, coarsely chopped
1 tbs baby capers, rinsed, drained, chopped
1 tbs white balsamic vinegar
Lemon wedges, to serve

1 Combine half each of the lemon juice, oil and dill in a shallow dish. Add the fish and turn to coat. Cover and set aside for 10 minutes to marinate.
2 Preheat a barbecue grill or chargrill pan on medium-high. Lightly spray the zucchini and squash with extra virgin olive oil. Grill the fish for 2 minutes each side or until cooked through. Set aside. Grill the zucchini and squash for 1 minute each side or until lightly charred and tender.
3 Place the zucchini and squash in a large bowl. Add the lentils, tomato, parsley, capers, vinegar and the remaining lemon juice, oil and dill. Gently toss to combine. Divide the salad among serving plates. Top with the fish and sprinkle with extra dill. Serve with lemon wedges to squeeze over.

COOK'S NOTE

If squash isn't available, use more zucchini or try capsicum. Serve with steamed wholemeal couscous or burghul, if you like.

NUTRITION (PER SERVE)

CALS	FAT	SAT FAT	PROTEIN	CARBS
287	9.6g	1.6g	31.6g	15.1g

★★★★★

I had a can of lentils at the back of the pantry, so thought I'd give this a go. Yum! So fresh and so fast! **VIOLAPARMESAN**

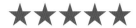

● EASY ○ QUICK ○ MAKE AHEAD ○ MEAT FREE ○ FAMILY FRIENDLY

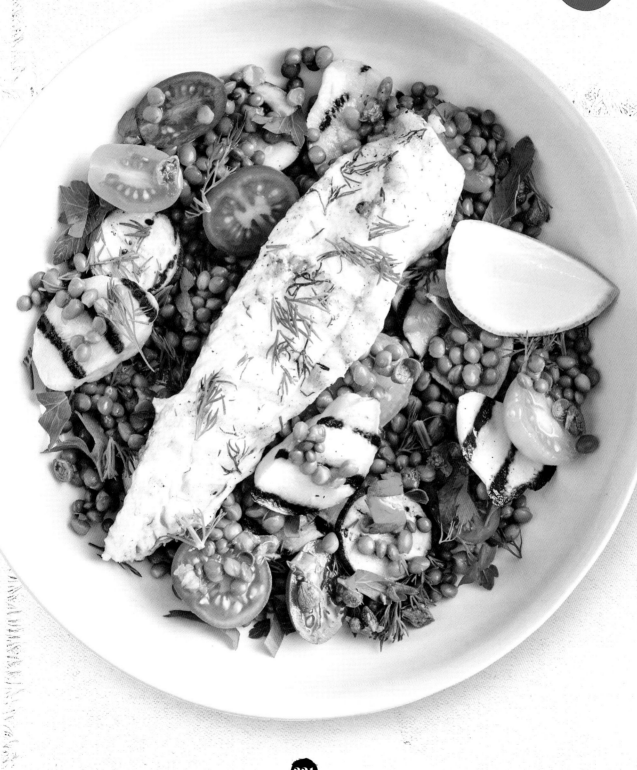

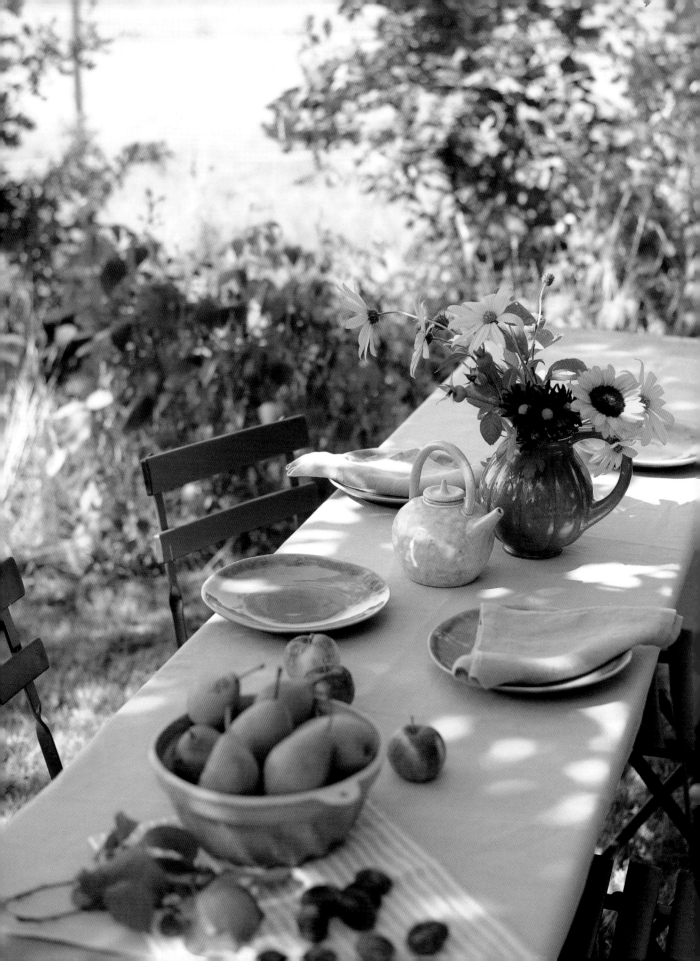

DESSERTS & TREATS

WHILE SWEETS ARE ONLY TO BE EATEN OCCASIONALLY IN A MEDITERRANEAN DIET, WHEN YOU DO, TREAT YOURSELF WITH HOMEMADE GOODIES. AIM FOR PLENTY OF FRUIT AND NUTS, AND USE NATURAL SWEETENERS.

Walnut & Zucchini BANANA BREAD

This loaf is full of wholesome ingredients and naturally sweetened with banana. The zucchini is a nutrient-rich way to keep the loaf moist.

SERVES 10 **PREP** 20 mins (+ cooling) **COOK** 1 hour 10 mins

235g (1½ cups) wholemeal spelt flour
50g (¼ cup) brown sugar
35g (⅓ cup) rolled oats
2 tbs chia seeds
2 tsp baking powder
1 tsp ground cinnamon
½ tsp bicarbonate of soda
20g walnut kernels
125ml (½ cup) buttermilk
60ml (¼ cup) light extra virgin
   olive oil
2 eggs
260g (1 cup) mashed ripe banana
1 small (about 120g) zucchini,
   coarsely grated
Honey and fresh low-fat ricotta,
   to serve (optional)

TOPPING
1 tbs rolled oats
1 tsp chia seeds
1 tsp brown sugar
½ tsp ground cinnamon

1 Preheat oven to 180°C/160°C fan forced. Grease and line the base and sides of a 9.5 x 19.5cm (base size) loaf pan, allowing the paper to overhang the sides.
2 To make the topping, combine all the topping ingredients in a small bowl.
3 Combine the flour, sugar, oats, chia seeds, baking powder, cinnamon and bicarb in a large bowl. Stir in the walnuts. Make a well in the centre.
4 Whisk together the buttermilk, oil and eggs in a jug then pour into the well. Add the banana and zucchini. Stir until just combined. Spoon the mixture into prepared pan. Scatter over the topping.
5 Bake for 1 hour 10 minutes or until a skewer inserted into the centre comes out clean. Set aside in pan for 10 minutes to cool slightly before transferring to a wire rack to cool completely.
6 Drizzle over honey and serve with a dollop of ricotta, if using.

COOK'S NOTE

Use this batter with a couple of tweaks to make muffins too! Search for 'healthy banana and zucchini muffins' on taste.com.au.

NUTRITION (PER SERVE)

CALS	FAT	SAT FAT	PROTEIN	CARBS
244	10g	1.6g	7g	30.4g

● EASY ○ QUICK ● MAKE AHEAD ● FAMILY FRIENDLY

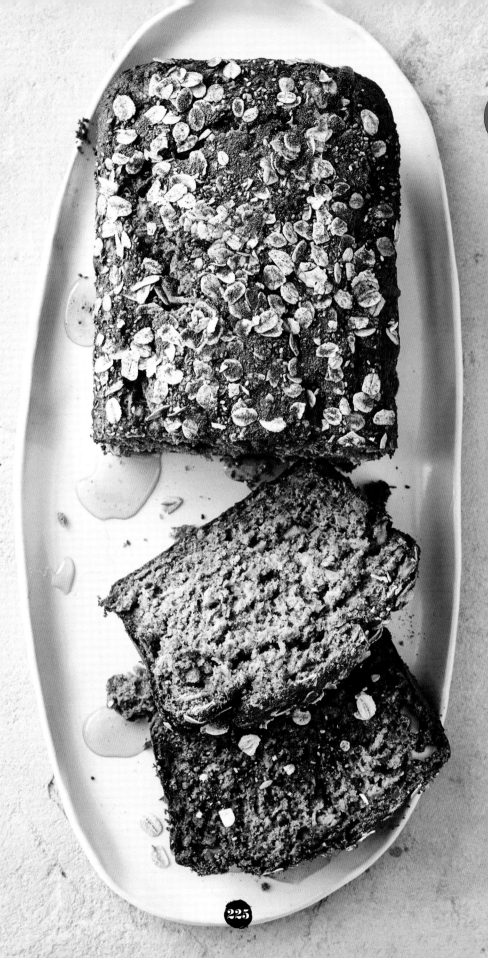

20+
*minutes
prep*

Filo & Roast
GRAPE PASTRIES

Believe it – these heavenly tarts aren't loaded with sugar!
We've used nuts, fresh fruit and spices for sweet, sweet satisfaction.

MAKES 16 **PREP** 30 mins **COOK** 35 mins

16 filo pastry sheets
30g (¼ cup) almond meal
2 tbs brown sugar
½ tsp ground cinnamon
¼ tsp ground cloves
150g seedless red grapes, halved
150g seedless green grapes, halved
25g (¼ cup) natural flaked almonds
Honey, to serve
Greek-style yoghurt, to serve
   (optional)

1 Preheat oven to 200°C/180°C fan forced. Line 2 large baking trays with baking paper.
2 Place the filo on a clean work surface. Cover with a dry tea towel then a damp tea towel (this will prevent it from drying out). Spray 1 filo sheet liberally with extra virgin olive oil. Fold in half lengthways. Starting at a long side, roll up about three-quarters of the way along then fold into a circle, tucking under the extra pastry and sealing the edges to make a small tart case. Place on one prepared tray. Repeat with the remaining filo to make 16 cases in total.
3 Combine the almond meal, sugar, cinnamon and cloves in a small bowl. Sprinkle the base of each tart case with the almond meal mixture. Top with the grapes. Scatter over the flaked almonds. Spray with oil. Bake for 30-35 minutes or until golden and crisp.
4 Drizzle over honey and serve warm or at room temperature with yoghurt, if using.

COOK'S NOTE

Use fruit that's in season – sliced plum, apple or pear, or halved strawberries are also delicious in these tarts.

NUTRITION (EACH)

CALS	FAT	SAT FAT	PROTEIN	CARBS
139	7.5g	1g	2.2g	15.4g

★★★★★

Roasted grapes are a revelation!

BAKINGSELFIES

● EASY ○ QUICK ○ MAKE AHEAD ● FAMILY FRIENDLY

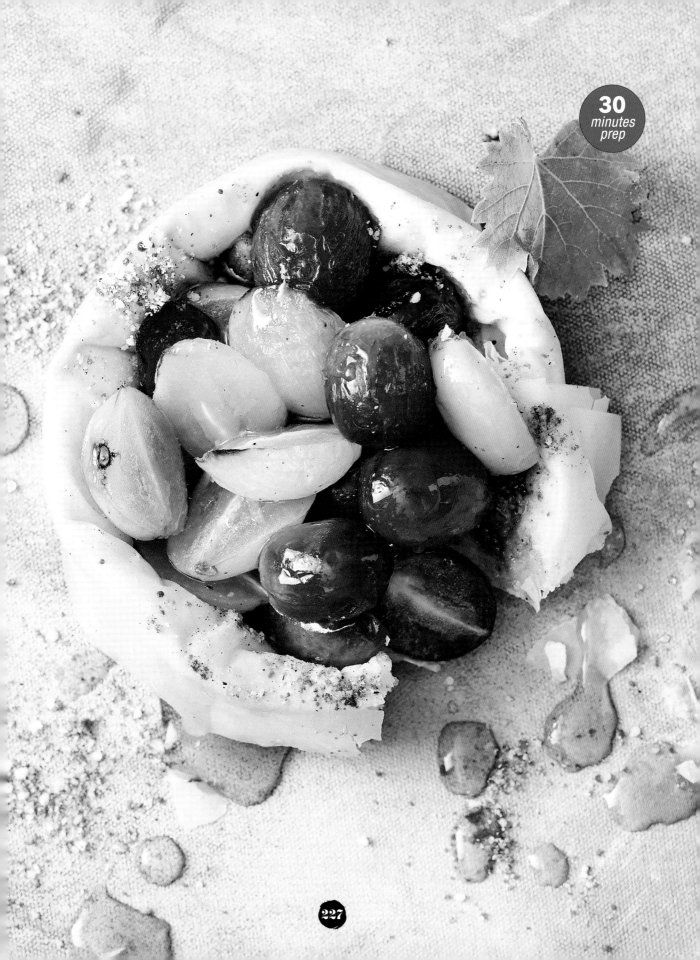

30
minutes
prep

Honey & Polenta
PEAR CAKE

Fold honey-caramelised pears into a better-for-you batter of polenta, almond meal and olive oil for afternoon tea perfection.

SERVES 10 **PREP** 15 mins (+ cooling) **COOK** 1 hour

1 tbs extra virgin olive oil,
   plus 125ml (½ cup) extra
60ml (¼ cup) honey, plus extra,
   warmed, to serve (optional)
3 pears, peeled, cored, cut into
   1cm pieces, plus 1 extra,
   unpeeled, cut into
   7 x 2mm-thick slices
85g (½ cup) buckwheat flour
80g fine polenta
80g (⅔ cup) almond meal
1½ tsp baking powder
3 eggs
2 tbs brown sugar
1 tsp vanilla extract
1 lemon, rind finely grated
1 tbs natural sliced almonds

1 Preheat oven to 180°C/160°C fan forced. Grease the base and side of a 22cm (base size) springform pan and double-line with baking paper.
2 Heat the oil and 2 tbs honey in a large non-stick frying pan over medium-high heat. Add the chopped pear. Cook, stirring occasionally, for 12 minutes or until golden. Transfer to a bowl.
3 Combine the flour, polenta, almond meal and baking powder in a separate bowl.
4 Use electric beaters to whisk the eggs, sugar, vanilla and remaining honey in a bowl for 5 minutes or until thickened and tripled in volume.
5 With the beaters on medium-low, slowly add the extra oil in a thin, steady stream until combined. Beat in the lemon rind. Use a large metal spoon to fold in the pear mixture and polenta mixture, in 2 alternating batches, until just combined. Pour into prepared pan. Top with extra sliced pear, arranging in the centre in a circle. Sprinkle with the almonds.
6 Bake, covering the pan with foil if over-browning, for 40-45 minutes or until a skewer inserted into the centre comes out clean. Set aside in the pan for 15 minutes to cool slightly before transferring to a wire rack to cool completely. Drizzle over extra warmed honey, if using.

COOK'S NOTE

This cake will keep up to 3 days in an airtight container.

NUTRITION (PER SERVE)

CALS	FAT	SAT FAT	PROTEIN	CARBS
332	20g	3g	6g	27g

● EASY   ○ QUICK   ● MAKE AHEAD   ● FAMILY FRIENDLY

15+ minutes prep

★★★★★
*Created an account to add a review because this recipe is that good!
Beautiful inside and out, adore it. Thank you.* **AKEELAH**

Cranberry & Orange
NO-BAKE SLICE

Slip one of these make-ahead bars in the school lunchbox or work bag for a fruit and nut snack everyone can get behind.

MAKES 20 **PREP** 20 mins (+ 4 hours chilling)

450g fresh medjool dates, pitted
125ml (½ cup) fresh orange juice
2 tsp finely grated orange rind
2 tbs honey
½ tsp ground cinnamon
1 tbs raw cacao powder
230g (1¼ cups) pepita and sunflower seed mix
360g (4 cups) rolled oats
55g (1 cup) coconut flakes
75g (½ cup) dried cranberries

1 Grease a 20 x 30cm (base size) slice pan. Line base and sides with baking paper, allowing the paper to overhang 2cm above the sides.
2 Place the dates, orange juice and rind, honey, cinnamon and cacao in a food processor. Add 150g (1 cup) seed mix, 180g (2 cups) oats and 45g (¾ cup) coconut. Process until finely chopped and the mixture comes together. Transfer to a bowl. Reserve 1 tbs cranberries then add the remaining cranberries and oats to the date mixture. Stir until well combined.
3 Press the mixture evenly into prepared pan. Sprinkle with the remaining seed mix, coconut and reserved cranberries, pressing firmly to secure. Place in the fridge for 4 hours or overnight until firm.
4 Cut into slices to serve.

COOK'S NOTE

Look for medjool dates in the fruit and veg section at the supermarket. Keep the slice in the fridge for up to 5 days.

NUTRITION (EACH)

CALS	FAT	SAT FAT	PROTEIN	CARBS
215	8.2g	2.2g	6g	27.4g

★★★★★

A batch of these sorted the fam's snack time all week!

FOODSLED

● EASY ○ QUICK ● MAKE AHEAD ● FAMILY FRIENDLY

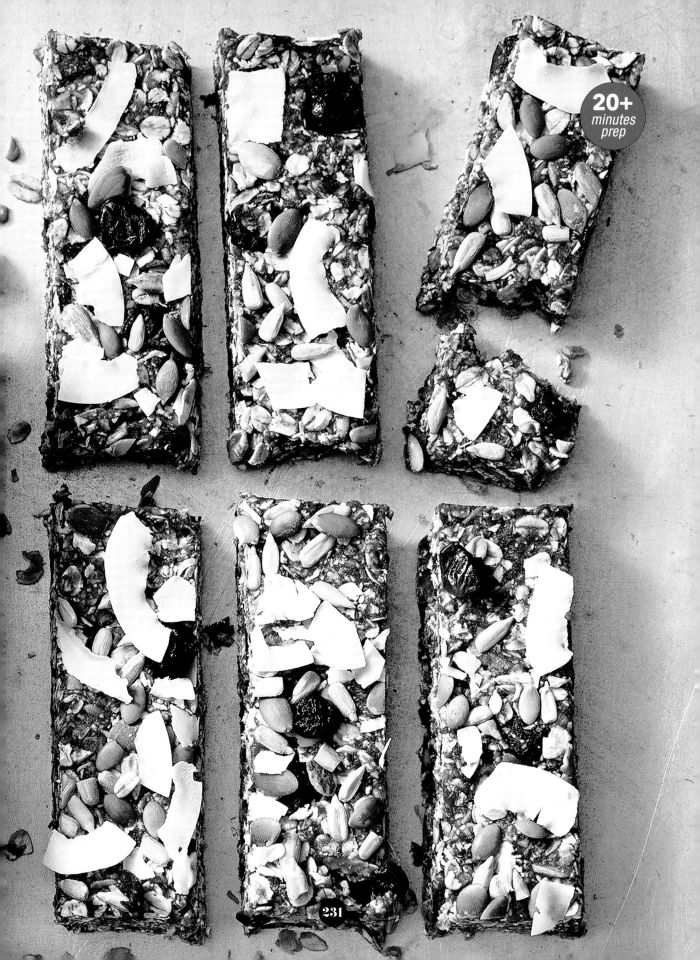

Toasty Spelt & Honey
BERRY CRUMBLE

Refined sugar free, this spelt and oat topping is sweet enough thanks to the honey- and vanilla-roasted fruit tucked underneath.

SERVES 6 **PREP** 15 mins (+ 5 mins cooling) **COOK** 1 hour

4 large pears, peeled, cored, cut into 1.5cm pieces
250g (2 cups) frozen raspberries
2 tbs honey
1 tsp vanilla bean paste
1 tbs wholemeal spelt flour
Greek-style yoghurt, to serve (optional)
CRUMBLE
90g (1 cup) rolled oats
45g (¼ cup) wholemeal spelt flour
½ tsp baking powder
2 tbs honey
1 tsp vanilla bean paste
1½ tbs olive oil spread

1 Preheat oven to 190°C/170°C fan forced. Lightly grease a 1L (4 cup) baking dish.
2 Combine the pear, raspberries, honey, vanilla and flour in a large bowl. Gently toss to combine. Transfer to prepared dish. Cover dish tightly with foil. Place on a large baking tray. Bake, stirring halfway through cooking, for 40 minutes or until the fruit is almost tender.
3 Meanwhile, make the crumble. Combine the oats, flour, baking powder, honey and vanilla in a bowl. Add the spread then use your fingertips to rub into the flour mixture until the mixture resembles coarse crumbs.
4 Scatter the crumble mixture over the fruit and bake, uncovered, for 20 minutes or until the topping is golden and the pear is tender. Set aside for 5 minutes to cool slightly. Top with yoghurt, if using.

COOK'S NOTE

Use any berries you like (fresh or frozen) in place of raspberries. Make up to 1 day ahead and keep in the fridge. Reheat in the oven.

NUTRITION (PER SERVE)

CALS	FAT	SAT FAT	PROTEIN	CARBS
282	4.7g	1g	4.1g	47g

★★★★★
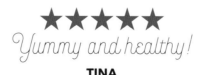
Yummy and healthy!
TINA

● EASY ○ QUICK ● MAKE AHEAD ● FAMILY FRIENDLY

15+
minutes
prep

★ ★ ★ ★ ★

Scrumptious, healthy dessert! I substituted the spelt flour with wholemeal. A hit with all the family. **SANDIOLA**

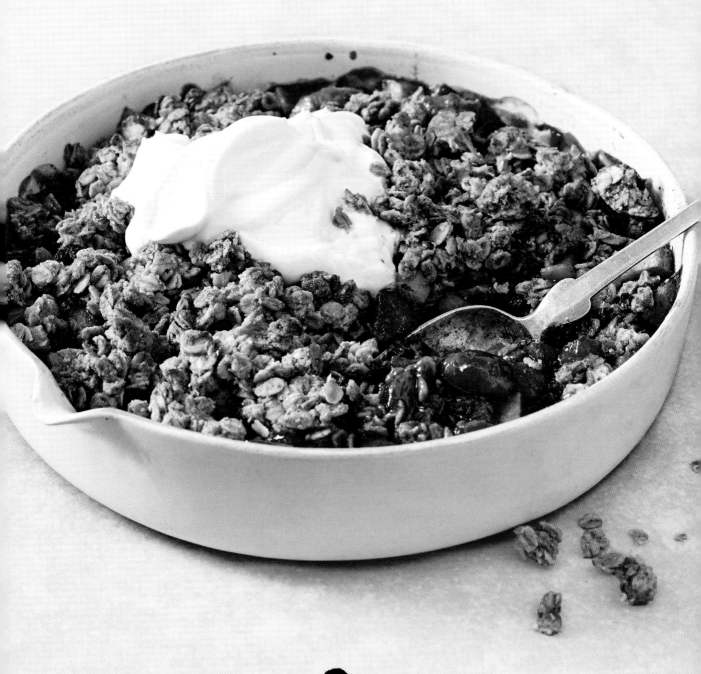

Little Orange POLENTA CAKES

Celebrate citrus with these muffin pan masterpieces!
Oranges are a treasure trove of nutrients and antioxidants.

MAKES 12 **PREP** 15 mins (+ cooling) **COOK** 20 mins

150g (1 cup) self-raising flour
90g (½ cup) polenta
80g pistachio kernels
1 tbs finely grated orange rind
2 eggs
80ml (⅓ cup) extra virgin olive oil
80ml (⅓ cup) honey, plus extra
    to serve
80ml (⅓ cup) fresh orange juice
2 small oranges (see note)

1 Preheat oven to 180°C/160°C fan forced. Grease a 12-hole 80ml (⅓ cup) muffin pan.
2 Place the flour, polenta, pistachios, orange rind, eggs, oil, honey and orange juice in a food processor. Process until the pistachios are finely chopped and the mixture is well combined. Divide the mixture among prepared muffin pan holes.
3 Peel and thinly slice the oranges into rounds (you'll need 12 slices in total). Place 1 orange slice on top of each pan hole. Bake for 18 minutes or until golden and just firm to the touch. Set aside in pan for 2 minutes to cool slightly before transferring to a wire rack.
4 Drizzle the tops with extra honey and set aside to cool. Serve warm or at room temperature.

COOK'S NOTE

Use navel oranges, if possible, as they are seedless. Alternatively, remove any seeds from orange slices before arranging on top of the cakes.

NUTRITION (EACH)

CALS	FAT	SAT FAT	PROTEIN	CARBS
223	10.5g	1.6g	4.4g	27.1g

★★★★★
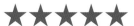
Lovely texture, easy to make. Great flavours. Sliced orange on top works well too. **JO**

● EASY   ○ QUICK   ○ MAKE AHEAD   ● FAMILY FRIENDLY

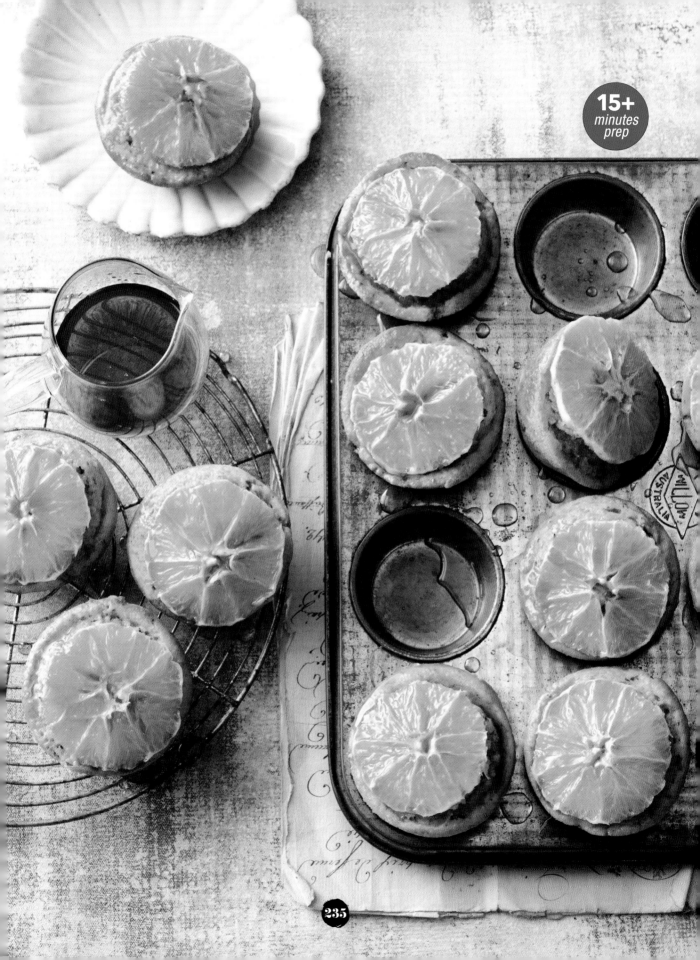

Seed Praline & Spiced
BAKED PEARS

This beauty has the cold-weather trifecta: fragrant baked pears, homemade labne and toasty seed crisps.

SERVES 4 **PREP** 20 mins (+ overnight draining & cooling) **COOK** 50 mins

500g low-fat Greek-style yoghurt
4 small (about 550g) beurre bosc pears, unpeeled, halved
300ml fresh orange juice
1 cinnamon stick
6 whole cloves
Large pinch of saffron
2½ tbs honey
1 tbs pistachio kernels, sliced
2 tsp sesame seeds
1 tsp poppy seeds
Large pinch of sea salt flakes

1 To make the labne, line a sieve with 2 layers of muslin cloth. (Alternatively, use 5 layers of paper towel.) Set prepared sieve over a bowl. Spoon the yoghurt into the sieve. Cover and place in the fridge overnight to drain the excess liquid from the yoghurt.
2 Preheat oven to 180°C/160°C fan forced. Place the pear, cut-side down, in a large roasting pan. Add the orange juice, cinnamon, cloves, saffron and 1 tbs honey. Cover with a piece of baking paper then cover the pan with foil. Bake for 30 minutes or until the pear is just tender. Uncover and turn the fruit and baste with the pan juices. Bake for a further 20 minutes or until tender. Set aside to cool.
3 Meanwhile, line a baking tray with baking paper. Combine the pistachios, sesame seeds, poppy seeds, salt and remaining honey in a bowl. Spoon onto prepared tray and spread slightly. Bake for 11-13 minutes or until dark golden. Set aside to cool completely before breaking into shards.
4 Spread some labne over each serving plate. Top with the pear, a drizzle of the pan juices and seed praline shards.

COOK'S NOTE

Store strained labne in an airtight container in the fridge for up to 2 days.

NUTRITION (PER SERVE)

CALS	FAT	SAT FAT	PROTEIN	CARBS
299	5g	2g	12g	42g

★★★★★

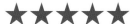

All the elements of this were delicious and worked so well together.

HARMONYPUFFIN

○ EASY   ○ QUICK   ○ MAKE AHEAD   ● FAMILY FRIENDLY

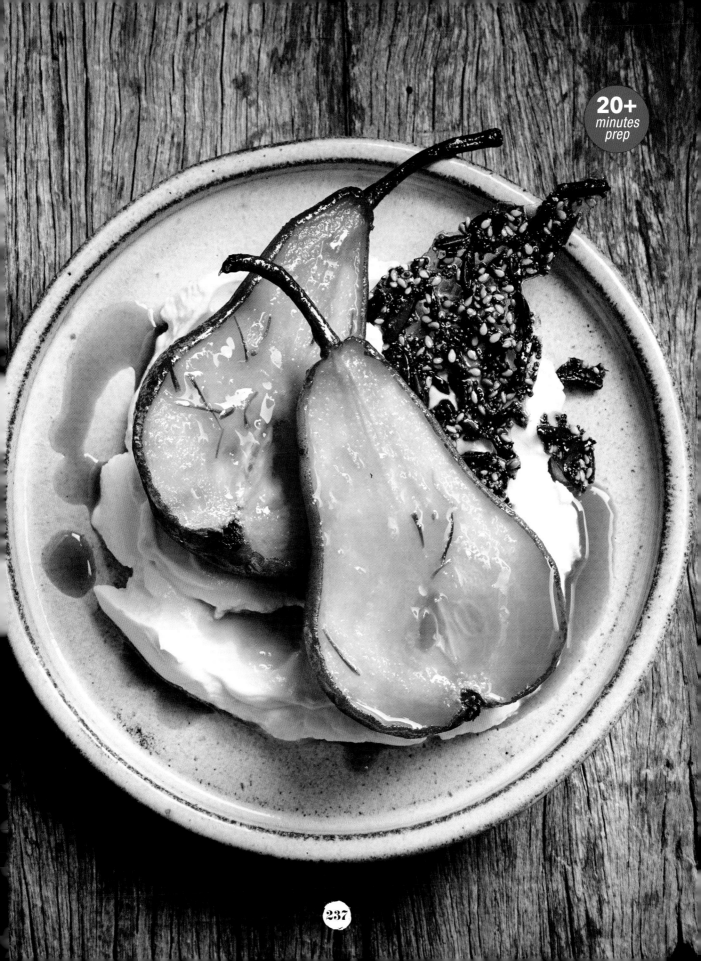

20+
minutes
prep

Honeyed Walnut
GINGER BISCUITS

Extra virgin olive oil – a staple of the Mediterranean diet – is so versatile and that's for sweets too. Use it in place of butter for light and moist biscuits.

MAKES 60 **PREP** 20 mins (+ 10 mins standing & cooling) **COOK** 30 mins

340g (2¼ cups) self-raising flour
1 tbs ground ginger
1 tsp baking powder
¼ tsp bicarbonate of soda
160ml (⅔ cup) extra virgin olive oil
2 tsp vanilla extract
1 egg, lightly whisked
2 tsp finely grated lemon rind
185ml (¾ cup) honey
60g (½ cup) coarsely chopped
   walnut kernels (see note)

1 Preheat oven to 180°C/160°C fan forced. Grease and line 3 large baking trays with baking paper.
2 Sift the flour, ginger, baking powder and bicarb into a large bowl. Make a well in the centre. Combine the oil, vanilla, egg, lemon rind and 125ml (½ cup) honey in a separate bowl then pour over the flour mixture. Mix until well combined. Set aside for 10 minutes to thicken slightly.
3 Place the walnuts on a plate. Roll 2 level teaspoonfuls of the mixture into a ball and flatten. Press 1 side into the walnuts. Place, walnut-side up, on a prepared tray. Repeat with the remaining mixture and walnuts. Bake, 1 tray at a time, for 10 minutes or until golden.
4 Meanwhile, combine the remaining honey and 2 tbs water in a small saucepan over medium heat. Cook for 2 minutes or until warmed and combined.
5 Brush the honey mixture over the hot biscuits. Set aside to cool completely before serving.

COOK'S NOTE

Use pecans or pistachios instead, if you prefer. Store biscuits in an airtight container for up to 5 days.

NUTRITION (EACH)

CALS	FAT	SAT FAT	PROTEIN	CARBS
64	3.4g	0.4g	0.8g	7.5g

★★★★★

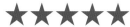 These are lovely with a cuppa. **DANI.BROUGHAM**

● EASY ○ QUICK ● MAKE AHEAD ● FAMILY FRIENDLY

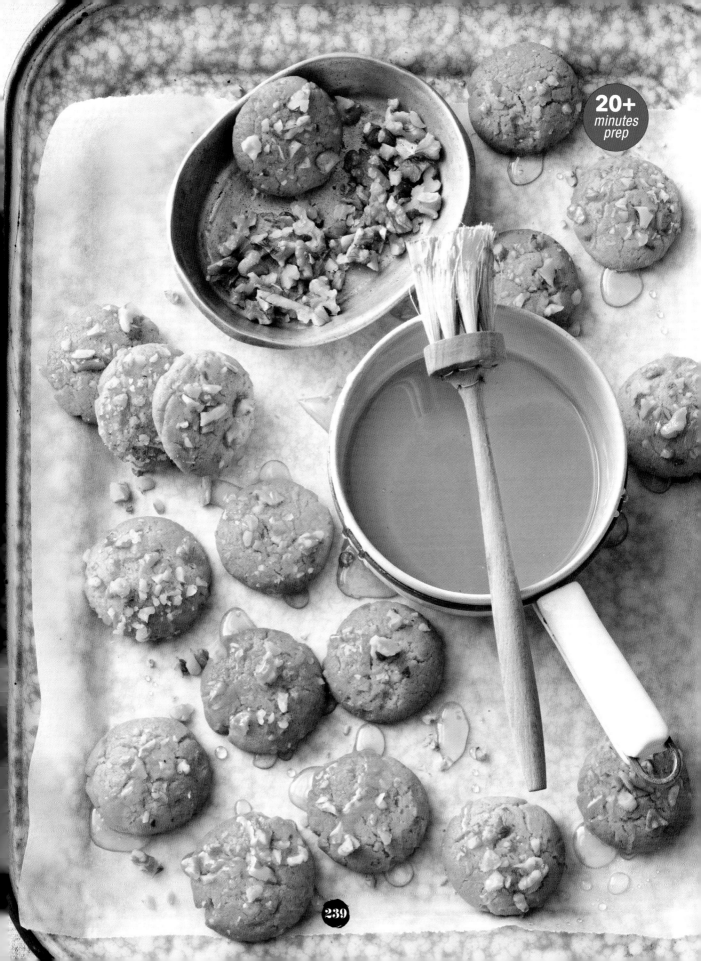

Rustic Spelt
APPLE TART

This free-form bake is much easier to make than
a traditional apple pie – the more rustic the better!

SERVES 8 **PREP** 30 mins (+ 1 hour resting) **COOK** 45 mins

175g white spelt flour
50g wholemeal spelt flour
¾ tsp ground cinnamon,
    plus extra to sprinkle
35g brown sugar
60ml (¼ cup) extra virgin
    olive oil, plus ½ tsp extra
90-100ml chilled water
3 small (about 410g) Granny Smith
    apples, peeled, quartered, cored
2 tsp fresh lemon juice
2 tbs apricot jam
Greek-style yoghurt, to serve
    (optional)

1 Place the flours, cinnamon and 1 tbs sugar in a large bowl. Stir to combine. Make a well in the centre. Pour in the oil in a slow steady stream, stirring with a fork, until incorporated and small lumps form. Add 90ml chilled water. Use a wooden spoon to stir until a tacky dough forms, adding more water if necessary.
2 Turn onto a lightly floured surface and briefly knead until just smooth. Shape the dough into a disc. Wrap in plastic wrap and place in the fridge for 1 hour to rest.
3 Meanwhile, preheat oven to 180°C/160°C fan forced. Cut each apple quarter into 4 thin slices. Place in a bowl. Add the lemon juice and 1 tbs of remaining sugar. Toss to coat.
4 Roll out the dough on a lightly floured sheet of baking paper to a 30cm disc. Carefully transfer the dough on the paper to a large baking tray. Spread with the jam, leaving a 3-4cm border around the edge. Top with the apple slices, arranging in concentric circles. Fold the pastry edge over the filling, roughly pleating. Brush the pastry edge with the extra oil. Sprinkle with the remaining sugar. Bake for 45 minutes or until golden and crisp. Set aside on the tray to cool.
5 Sprinkle with extra cinnamon and serve at room temperature with yoghurt, if using.

COOK'S NOTE

Spelt flour is made from spelt, a type of wheat and one of the ancient grains. It is thought to be easier to digest than regular flour. Use plain flour if unavailable.

NUTRITION (PER SERVE)

CALS	FAT	SAT FAT	PROTEIN	CARBS
219	7.5g	1.2g	3.7g	33.5g

● EASY ○ QUICK ○ MAKE AHEAD ● FAMILY FRIENDLY

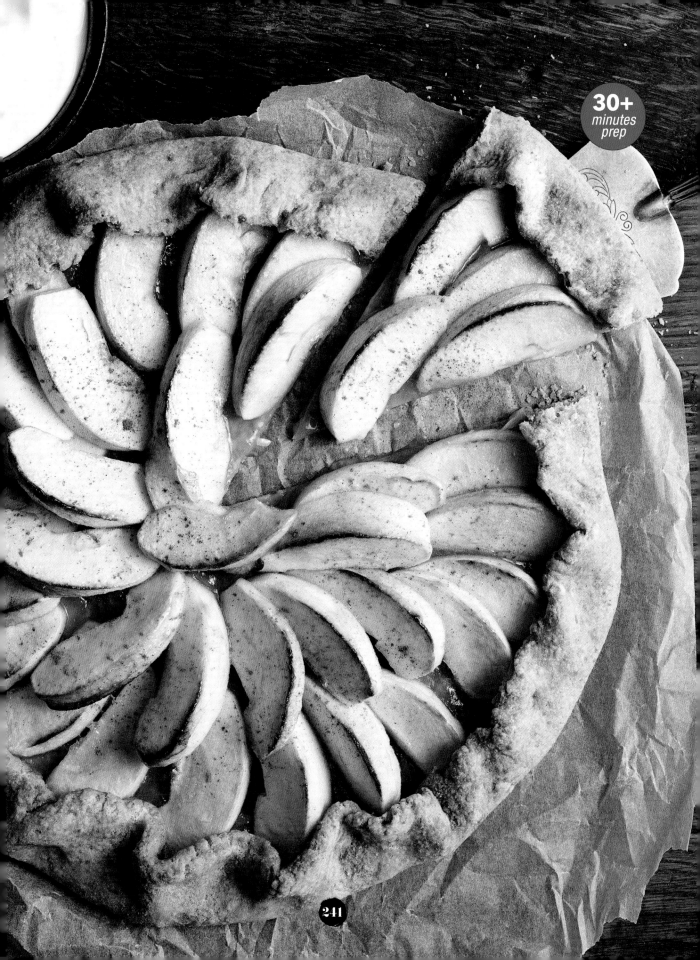

Choc-Banana
CHIA PUDDING

Choc-a-block with chia, this dessert pot tastes indulgent while you also enjoy the anti-inflammatory benefits of all those extra omega-3s!

SERVES 4 **PREP** 5 mins (+ overnight chilling)

4 bananas
1 tbs cocoa powder
500ml (2 cups) skim milk
80g (½ cup) white chia seeds
2 tbs natural peanut butter

1 Peel 2 bananas. Place in a bowl with the cocoa. Use a fork to mash. Stir in the milk. Add the chia and stir until combined. Cover and place in the fridge overnight to thicken.
2 Peel and thinly slice the remaining bananas. Spoon the chia pudding into serving glasses. Top with the sliced banana and peanut butter.

NUTRITION (PER SERVE)

CALS	FAT	SAT FAT	PROTEIN	CARBS
308	13.3g	1.9g	12.2g	29.7g

COOK'S NOTE

While this looks and tastes like a delicious dessert, you can also have it for brekky. Prep the night before so you can grab and go! Add berries too, if you like.

★ ★ ★ ★ ★

I had all the makings of this already. It was yum!

FANCY FOODIE

● EASY ● QUICK ● MAKE AHEAD ● FAMILY FRIENDLY

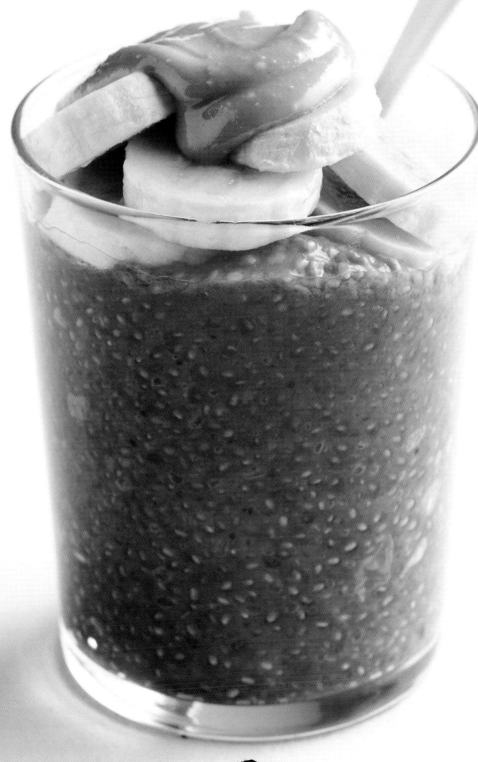

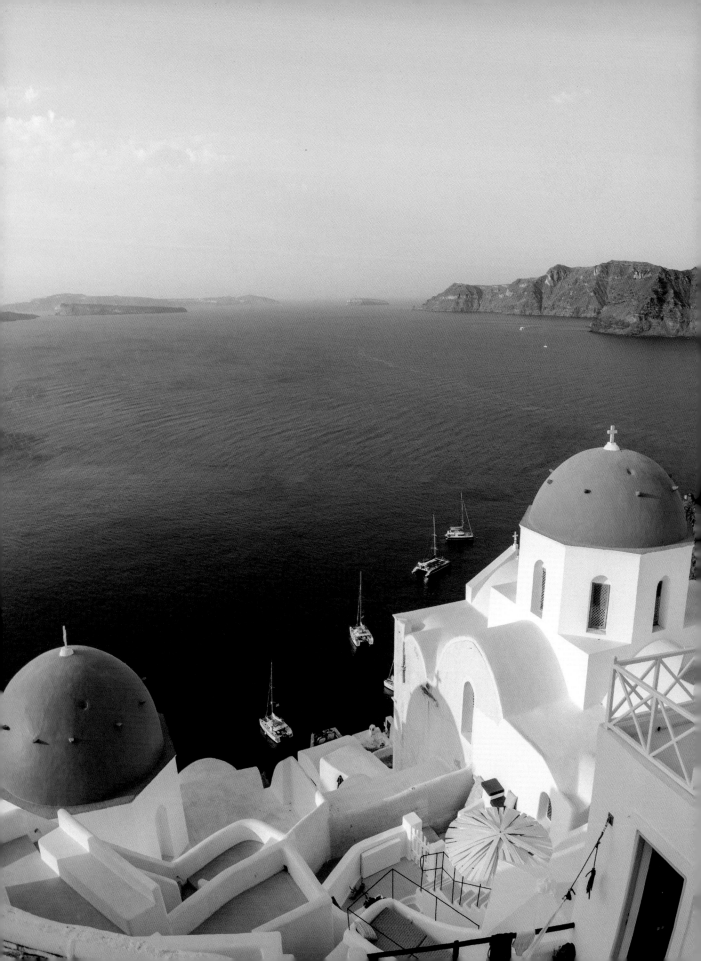

INDEX

USE OUR HANDY THREE-PART INDEX TO FIND
EVERY RECIPE – VIA ALPHABETICAL ORDER,
EASY KEY GUIDE OR INGREDIENT.

ALPHABETICAL INDEX

Here's a list of every recipe in this book to make it easier to find the ones you want to make again and again.

INDEX BY KEY GUIDE

INDEX BY INGREDIENT

CREDITS

editor-in-chief Brodee Myers
executive editor & book editor Alex McDivitt
food director Michelle Southan
creative director Harmony Southern
book art director Chi Lam
book food editor Tracy Rutherford
nutrition editor Chrissy Freer
editorial coordinator Xenia Taylor

managing director – food and travel Fiona Nilsson

HarperCollins*Publishers* Australia
publishing director Brigitta Doyle
head of Australian non-fiction Helen Littleton
project editor Shannon Kelly

CONTRIBUTORS

Recipes Alison Adams, Claire Brookman, Kim Coverdale, Chrissy Freer, Amira Georgy, Louise Keats, Kathy Knudsen, Cathie Lonnie, Gemma Luongo, Liz Macri, Lucy Nunes, Miranda Payne, Kerrie Ray, Tracy Rutherford, Jo-Anne Woodman, Katrina Woodman, Sophia Young

Photography Guy Bailey, Ben Dearnley, Vanessa Levis, Andy Lewis, Nigel Lough, Amanda McLauchlan, Mark O'Meara, Al Richardson, Jeremy Simons, Brett Stevens, Andrew Young, Craig Wall

Illustration Kat Chadwick

Additional photography Getty Images

HarperCollins*Publishers*
Australia • Brazil • Canada • France • Germany • Holland • India • Italy
Japan • Mexico • New Zealand • Poland • Spain • Sweden • Switzerland
United Kingdom • United States of America

HarperCollins acknowledges the Traditional Custodians of the land upon which we live and work, and pays respect to Elders past and present.

First published on Gadigal Country in Australia in 2024
by HarperCollins*Publishers* Australia Pty Limited
ABN 36 009 913 517
harpercollins.com.au

A catalogue record for this book is available from the National Library of Australia

ISBN 978 1 4607 6575 3 (paperback)
ISBN 978 1 4607 1741 7 (ebook)

Colour reproduction by Splitting Image Colour Studio, Wantirna, Victoria
Printed and bound in China

8 7 6 5 4 3 2 1   24 25 26 27 28

THANK YOU

We'd like to thank everyone
who contributed to this book: our foodies,
photographers, stylists, editors, designers
and digital team. Each recipe is a result of
amazing dedication and teamwork.
A shout out to our nutritionist,
Chrissy Freer, for her wisdom and guidance –
from recipe selection to nutrition and
everything in between!
A huge thank you to Brigitta Doyle
and Helen Littleton, our partners at
HarperCollins. We're very thankful
for your expertise and support.
And lastly, a thank you to … you, our
audience. Thousands of passionate cooks
visit our site every day to plan, cook and
share reviews, ratings and tips. We love
hearing about your joy for cooking and the
gusto with which you make our recipes,
so keep those reviews coming!

Want more healthy?

...ut healthy at your fingertips with the app from Australia's #1 food site, taste.com.au. Every taste ...ipe is here, including 7,500 deliciously nutritious dishes that you, your family and friends will love.

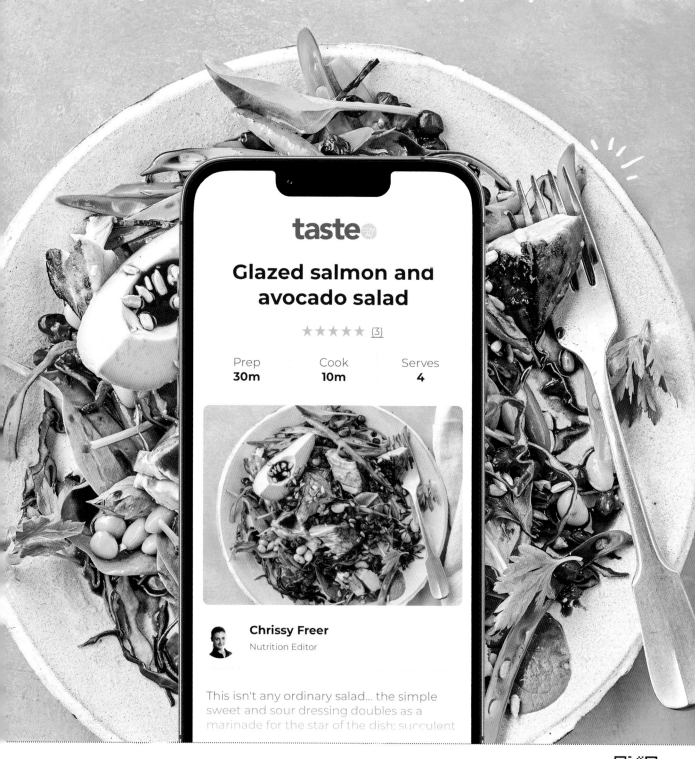

taste.com.au

Glazed salmon and avocado salad

★★★★★ (3)

Prep	Cook	Serves
30m	10m	4

Chrissy Freer
Nutrition Editor

This isn't any ordinary salad... the simple
sweet and sour dressing doubles as a
marinade for the star of the dish; succulent